CW00705840

BLOOD PF

Etiology and Homeopathic Management

Dr. N. K. Banerjee, M.Sc., M.H.M.S.

Principal, Bengal Allen Homeopathic Medical College and Hospital, Calcutta;
Formerly, President, General Council and State Faculty of Homeopathic Medicine, Government of West Bengal;
Member, Homeopathic Rural Aid Committee and Sub-Committee of Drugs Technical Advisory Board, Govt. of India; Vice-president, Homeo. Pharmaceutical Chemists' Association, West Bengal; President, Indian Homeopathic Association, and Author of 'Practice of Medicine, with Homeopathic Therapeutics' and 'Realistic Materia Medica with Therapeutical Repertory, etc.

NEW REVISED AND ENLARGED EDITION

B. Jain Publishers (P) Ltd.

An ISO 9001 : 2000 Certified Company
USA – Europe – India

BLOOD PRESSURE

New Revised & Enlarged Edition: 2007
6th Impression: 2010

Published by Kuldeep Jain for
B. JAIN PUBLISHERS (P) LTD.
An ISO 9001 : 2000 Certified Company
1921/10, Chuna Mandi, Paharganj, New Delhi 110 055 (INDIA)
Tel.: +91-11-4567 1000 • *Fax:* +91-11-4567 1010
Email: info@bjain.com • *Website:* **www.bjain.com**

Printed in India

ISBN: 978-81-319-1075-7

Dedicated

to the

Members of the Healing Profession

Preface to the New Edition

In this Edition the whole text has been fully revised and corrected. Some additions here and there were found necessary to be incorporated to enhance further the practical utility of the Book and they have been embodied.

N.K. Banerjee

Preface to the New Edition

This Monograph on "Blood Pressure" is my humble attempt to give a lucid and comprehensive treatment of the subject within the limited space at my disposal. I have all through aimed at clarity of exposition and have scrupulously avoided all discussions of a purely academic or controversial nature, which is appropriate for a more ambitious undertaking.

It is undeniable that, the proper understanding of the pathological state is a condition precedent to the rational management of the hypertensive and to the just evaluation of the changes in the blood pressure readings in terms of prognosis. Therefore, the chief aim of this book has been to explain the mechanism by which normal blood pressure is maintained and the factors that tend to alter the tension in health and disease. On the basis of such explanation, an idea could be formed of the effects, which those factors have, on the life and longevity of the subject and the steps needed for the rational treatment of the case in hand.

I do not pretend to claim any great originality for this treatise. As a matter of fact, I have consulted and drawn heavily upon various authoritative books on the subject and, therefore, I owe a large obligation to those authorities. What I have sought to do in this treatise is to present the complex, if not confusing, knowledge in a more simple, compact and digestible form, particularly to the noviciate for facility of consumption and assimilation.

The part dealing with the Homeopathic Repertory and the remedial treatment on the basis of symptomatology has been written with a great deal of care and deep consideration. The chapter at the end 'Resume of the Therapeutics of Blood Pressure', may be found to be of great advantage to busy practitioners in acute and emergent cases.

My labour would be amply rewarded if this book proves helpful to the profession, to which it is dedicated. I shall receive with gratitude any suggestions which the profession may like to offer for its further improvement.

N. K. Banerjee

Contents

I. Introduction

By the term BLOOD PRESSURE people are inclined to think of a serious disease of modern civilisation. Blood pressure does not, in the strict sense of the term, mean a disease at all. It is essential for life, and every living man or woman carries some degree of blood pressure.

In certain pathological states, the blood pressure rises above the normal figure, sometimes reaching such heights as to become a source of imminent danger to life, but a sign or manifestation of a pathological process just as fever is not a disease but measurable external index of an internal malady. It might be said in consonance both with reason and science, that the rise of blood pressure is a CONSERVATIVE or COMPENSATORY process by which adequate circulation of blood is maintained in the tissues in spite of increased resistance or obstruction to the flow of blood. If the blood pressure would fail to rise while the obstruction to the flow of blood be increasing, the inevitable result would be death from failure of circulation. To bring the analogy closer between fever and increased blood pressure, it may be asserted that a rise of blood pressure is a necessary evil to support life in adverse circumstances of blood-flow as much as fever is an unpleasant reaction but, nevertheless, conducive to the body to fight out the invading disease. But both fever and blood pressure should remain within safe limits, and every effort should be made to reduce them when they assume alarming proportions. It must be born in mind that a drastic reduction of fever or blood pressure by drugs is fraught with grave consequences, and should by no means be attempted. Removal of the cause to which the body reacts by fever or increased blood pressure is the ideal method of treatment.

High blood pressure, which is also known as HYPERTENSION, seems to be commoner in modern times than in the good old days. It cannot be denied that the modern civilisation has brought in its trail a great deal of adverse factors tending to raise blood pressure. Intensive struggle for existence associated with continual anxiety, greedy ambition, artificial methods of living, want of faith in religion, intemperance, irregular hours, adulterated and unwholesome food, and many vices peculiar to modern civilisation do undoubtedly play important parts in its causation. Moreover, with the discovery of the Sphygmomanometer, the detection of raised blood pressure has become an easy affair and, therefore, more cases are brought to the notice of the profession today than before. However, it cannot be contended that hypertension was a rarity in the good old days, since apoplexy (Sannyash Roga) has been dealt with in the medical treatises of the Ayurvedic System of Medicine.

II. Circulation

In order to appreciate the importance of blood pressure, a thorough understanding of the **CIRCULATION** is requisite. Circulation means a continual out-flow of blood from the heart along certain channels called the arteries and the capillaries and then back to the heart itself through the veins. Or, in other words, the blood-stream flows round and round the same course in a cyclic fashion, without pause or intermission.

The POWER, which keeps the blood moving continually, is jointly supplied by the heart and the elasticity of the arterial wall. This power is needed to push the blood forward by overcoming the resistance to the flow of blood as given by the small arteries called the arterioles and the capillaries. For the circulation to be continual, both the power and the resistance are essential. This will be explained later in this treatise.

The Heart

The heart is a muscular pump, situated obliquely in the chest-cavity between the lungs, so that the major part of it lies to the left of the mid-sternal line. It is divided by a musculo-membranous partition into the RIGHT and the LEFT sides. Each side presents an upper small chamber called the AURICLE, and a lower larger chamber known as the VENTRICLE. The right chambers are concerned entirely with ARTERIAL or pure oxygenated blood. The phase of contraction of the heart is called the SYSTOLE, while the phase of relaxation and rest is known as the DIASTOLE.

Venous or impure blood is poured into the right auricle by the Superior and the Inferior Vene Cava, the two venous terminal trunks, the former bringing the impure blood from the head, neck and upper limbs, while the latter draining the impure blood from the rest of the body. The filling of the auricle is helped by the suction-action of the expanding auricle after contraction, as well as by the increased negative pressure produced inside the chest during inspiration.

The right auricle communicates with the right ventricle by means of a door guarded by a valve

(TRICUSPID), which would allow only a one-way traffic, permitting the flow of blood from the auricle into the ventricle, and not in the opposite direction. When the ventricles relax, the A.V. valves (auriculo-ventricular valves) open, and by contraction of the auricles, the auricular blood rapidly rushes into the ventricles completing the ventricular filling. Here the auricular systole ends and is followed by the ventricular systole. When the auricular systole occurs, the mouths of the Superior and the Inferior Vene Cava are shut by the contraction of the circular muscular fibres encircling their mouths, so that the blood cannot flow back into them.

The right ventricle, having received venous blood from the right auricle, pumps it through the PULMONARY ARTERY into the lungs for oxygenation of the blood and for washing out its carbon dioxide in the breath. When the right ventricle contracts to drive the blood into the lungs, the tricuspid valve closes to prevent its backward flow, while the SEMILUNAR valve, guarding the mouth of the pulmonary artery, is forced open to allow the passage of blood to the right and the left lungs via the right and the left branches of the pulmonary artery.

In the lungs, the pulmonary arteries divide and subdivide into smaller and smaller braches till a network of very fine vessele (CAPILLARIES) is produced, their walls being so thin as to allow gaseous exchanges, the hemoglobin of the blood combines with the oxygen from the inspired air and the carbon dioxide of the blood is got rid of in the expired air. These capillaries unite with each other and make fine veins, which in turn unite with each other to make bigger veins. Thus, the process goes on till four PULMONARY VEINS are formed, two for each lung. These veins open into the left auricle by separate openings, through which the oxygenated blood from the lungs is received into the left auricle.

The left auricle, like the right one, communicates with the left ventricle by means of a door guarded by a valve (BICUSPID OR MITRAL), to allow a one-way traffic.

The left ventricle receives the oxygenated blood from the left auricle, exactly in the same way as the right ventricle receives its blood from the right auricle. When the left ventricle contracts, the mitral valve closes and the AORTIC VALVE, guarding the mouth of the aorta, opens and the blood flows forwards into the aorta.

The auricles contract together just before the simultaneous contraction of both the ventricles. After the auricular systole, the auricles relax and continue in that state of diastole, during ventricular contraction, as well as for most of the period of ventricular rest (diastole). The events from the beginning of one auricular systole to the beginning of the next constitute the CARDIAC CYCLE.

The heart beats 72 times per minute on the average in a healthy young man at rest. On that basis each cardiac cycle takes 0.8 second.

Auricular systole – 0.05   sec. ⎫
Auricular diastole – 0.75   sec. ⎭   = 0.8 sec.

Ventricular systole – 0.3   sec. ⎫
Ventricular diastole – 0.5   sec. ⎭   = 0.8 sec.

Any increase of the heart rate is always at the expense of the rest period of the heart, that is, the diastole.

The Arterial System

The system of tubes through which the blood flows away from the heart to the tissues is known as the ARTERIAL SYSTEM. There is a parent trunk called the AORTA, which rises from the left ventricle. From the Aorta, big branches are given off. From these big branches further braches arise. This braching process goes on till very small arteries called the ARTERIOLES are produced.

Beyond these arterioles capillary networks are formed, through which gaseous and other exchanges take place between the blood and the tissues. The whole arterial system bears a close resemblance to a tree with its trunk, branches, twigs and leaves.

The arteries are not rigid tubes. The elastic tissue preponderates in the large arteries, while the muscular tissue is most developed in the medium and small arteries. The capillaries have very thin transparent walls made of a single layer of endothelial cells which are capable of contraction. On the walls of the capillaries are found a peculiar type of cells called the ROUGET CELLS, having thread like branching processes forming a network around the capillaries. These cells, by their contraction and relaxation, bring about alterations of the size of the capillaries.

The muscular tissue of the arteries and the arterioles, which is of the plain or involuntary variety, as well as the capillaries are under the control of the autonomic nervous system, comprising of VASOCONSTRICTOR and VASODILATOR mechanisms. The Vasodilator mechanism comes into play to dilate the arterioles and the capillaries according to requirements. Therefore, the peripheral resistance to blood flow may increase or decrease according to the degree of vasoconstriction or vasodilatation, which is determined by the autonomic nervous system.

The velocity of the flow of blood is not the same in all the tubes of the arterial system. The bigger the artery the faster is the flow. In the Aorta, the blood flows at the rate of a foot per second, while in the capillaries the flow is an inch per minute. Or, in other words, the arterioles and the capillaries constitute the peripheral resistance, which increase or decrease according to the state and degree of contraction or relaxation of the arterioles and the capillaries.

The Venous System

The capillaries unite to from small veins, which unite again to form larger ones. The process of forming larger and larger veins continue till two large venous trunks come into existence, namely, the Superior and the Inferior vene cava. Except in very minute veins and in those veins which are not subjected to muscular pressure, there are valves, usually found in pairs, to guide the flow of blood, by preventing its backward flow, from the periphery towards the heart.

The Blood Flow

We know that blood flows continually without pause or intermission. How that is possible when it is admitted that the heart pours blood into the arteries intermittently, the blood being sent in only during the contraction of the heart and not during its relaxation ? A simple experiment will explain as to how the flow could

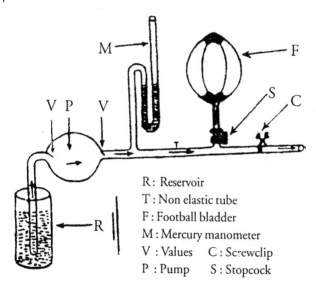

R : Reservoir
T : Non elastic tube
F : Football bladder
M : Mercury manometer
V : Values   C : Screwclip
P : Pump   S : Stopcock

P is a pump which, when worked by hand, sucks a fluid from the reservoir R, and forces it into the tube T on account of the valves V.

T is a non-elastic tube, having attachment to the pump at one end and screw-clip C at the other, by means of which the out-flow of fluid past C can be increased or decreased.

F is a football bladder, and therefore elastic, which is filled with fluid and connected to the tube T. S is a stop-cock which can connect or disconnect the fluids in T and F. M is a mercury manometer, to measure the pressure of fluid in the tube T during the contraction and relaxation of the pump P.

If S is closed and C fully open and the pump P is worked by hand, the fluid will flow out of C intermittently in coincidence with the squeeze. Very little force is required to empty the pump, and consequently, the Mano-meter M will show a small rise of pressure during squeezing.

If now C is tightened, or in other words, the reistance to the flow is increased, more force would be required to empty the pump P. But all the same, the flow at C will remain intermittent. The Manometer M will show greater rise of pressure when the pump is squeezed.

If now S is opened to establish connection between the fluids in the rigid tube T and the elastic bladder F, the working of the pump entails less force because, the fluid which cannot escape past C enters and distends the bladder F. Here the flow at C is no longer intermittent but constant because, during the filling of the pump, the distended elastic bladder recoils on the fluid in F and propels it outwards through C, since it can not go backwards into P on account of the valve V. The Manometer M shows less fluctuation in pressure; that is, the difference between the pressures at M during the contraction and relaxation of the pump is not so great after S is opened. The more C is tightened, the more would be the difference between the pressures during contraction and relaxation of the pump.

If the pump fills fully, the flow at C will be greater than if it fills partially. That is, the supply of fluid to the pump from the reservoir R determines the output from the pump, which, in turn, determines the fluid pressure as well as the volume of fluid flowing past C.

Therefore, for the flow to be continuous at C, four factors are required: -

(a) Regular and proper supply of fluid to the pump from R,

(b) Intermittent action of the pump P,

(c) Elastic recoil of the bladder F pressing the fluid out when the pump is filling,

(d) Resistance to the flow by tightening C.

These are exactly the factors which maintain a constant flow of blood, irrespective of the fact whether the heart is in a state of systole or diastole.

The Superior and the Inferior vene cava form the reservoir from which the pump heart is filled. Each ventricle pumps about 3 ounces of blood, the right ventricle sending it to the lungs and the left ventricle sending it into the already full Aorta, at each contraction.

The Aorta is distended by the extra three ounces of blood forced into it by the ventricular power. When the ventricle goes into diastole, the elastic wall of the Aorta recoils on its column of blood, and tends to flow it back into the ventricle. On account of the valve guarding the mouth of the Aorta, the blood can not flow back into the heart but flows forwards towards the periphery.

The peripheral resistance is afforded by the arterioles and capillaries, which are in a constant tonic state due to the action of the vasoconstrictor mechanism.

Blood Pressure

The pressure which the blood exerts on the wall of the vessels is called BLOOD PRESSURE. During the contraction of the ventricle, (SYSTOLE) it is the maximum, while when the ventricle is filling, (DIASTOLE) it is the minimum. The maximum pressure of blood in an artery is called SYSTOLIC PRESSURE, as it coincides with the systole of the ventricle. The minimum pressure in an artery is called the DIASTOLIC PRESSURE, as it coincides with the diastole of the ventricle. The difference between the maximum and the minimum pressures is known as the PULSE PRESSURE. It is the pulse pressure which keeps the blood moving constantly.

The blood pressure is not of the same degree in all the vessels. It is much more in those arteries which are nearer to the heart than in those which are further away from the heart.

In the BRACHIAL ARTERY, the artery of choice for taking blood pressure reading, the systolic pressure in a healthy young man at rest is about 120 *mm Hg*, while the blood pressure in the capillaries is between 20 to 10 *mm Hg*. In the veins the blood pressure of the elbow held at the level of the right auricle is only between 2 to

10 *mm.* of *Hg.* The table below gives an idea of the variation of blood pressure in different vessels.

Blood Pressure in Different Vessels

		Systolic	Diastolic
Left ventricle	...	150	
Aorta	...	150	100
Brachial artery	...	120	80
Radial artery	...	100	70
Arterioles	...	80	60
Capillaries	...	20	20
Small veins	...	15	15
Femoral vein	...	20	
Inferior vene cava	...	3	

Recording the Blood Pressure in Man

The blood pressure in man is recorded by the Sphygmomanometer. There are two types of Sphygmomanometer, the MERCURY COLUMN INSTRUMENT and the DIAL INSTRUMENT. The mercury column instrument is more in use, because the instrumental error in blood pressure reading is nil or negligible. However old the instrument might be, it remains more or less dependable since it is the height of the mercury column which determines the pressure. The dial instrument is liable to more instrumental error partiuclarly when old, since the correct reading depends upon the correct resistance of the spring, which is likely to be undermined with age. If the dial instrument is new, it is as reliable as the other.

Procedure

(a) The Auscultatory Method

The patient should be sitting in a comfortable and relaxed position, with his arm resting on a table ; or he should lie down on his back with the arm comfortably stretched out on the bed.

The arm-band containing an elastic bag is wrapped round the arm, so that the lower edge of the band lies about an inch above the bend of the elblow. The elastic bag is now connected with the Syphygmomanometer and air is pumped into the bag to distend it, and thereby to compress the brachial artery and obliterate the radial pulse. The chest piece of the binaural stethoscope is placed on the brachial artery below the arm band, to listen to any click or murmur. By means of the escape valve which is attached to the pump, air is gradually relased from the elastic bag to reduce its pressure on the brachial artery, as is shown by the descending mercury column in the

Sphygmomanometer.

When the pressure is being reduced, five phases are differentiated as follows:

The first phase – A distinct click is detected to appear at a certain point, synchronising with the heart beat. This point is read off on the Manometer as the systolic pressure, and indicates the force of the heart which is just suffcient for the transmission of the pulse through the brachial artery in that state of compression. This click is heard a trifle earlier than the return of the radial pulse.

The second phase – The click changes to a murmur with a click or a murmur alone.

The third phase – It is ushered in by a loud tap.

The fourth phase – The loud tap suddenly changes to a dull tone. At this point the diastolic pressure is read off on the Manometer.

The fifth phase – The dull tone completely disappears and no sound is heard.

There are some, who belive that the disappearance of the sound, the fifth phase, is the diastolic point. Except in very high blood pressure cases, the difference between the 4th and the 5th phases is only about 4 to 6 *mm Hg* in many instances. But sometimes, especially in the young adults, the difference may be even 30 *mm Hg*. Therefore, to take the abolition of the sound as the diastolic point would lead to serious error.

In some cases of Hypertension, particularly where the blood pressure is high, the second phase of murmur may not be heard at all. This possibility of missing the second phase should be borne in mind, otherwise serious error may be committed by accepting the appearance of the tap of the third phase as the systolic point.

(b) The Palpatory Method

The blood pressure may be recorded by feeling the pulse. The auscultatory or the auditory method, as described above, is the method of choice today. However, the palpatory method is still practised by some and therefore, it is given below.

The patient sits or lies, as in the first method, and the arm-band is wrapped round the arm as usual. Air is pumped into the bag which presses on the brachial artery. The mercury column not only rises in the Manometer but also oscillates with the brachial pulse. As the pressure in the bag is being raised, the oscillations increase and become greatest at a particular point. This point of maximal pulsation indicates the diastolic point. With the continued rise of pressure in the bag, the oscillations diminish and finally stop and the pulse is no longer to be felt at the wrist. The height of the mercury column should now be read off on the Manometer in order to get the systolic pressure.

The Average Normal Blood Pressure

It should always be borne in mind that the blood pressure of an individual is not a fixed entity. Normally, it may vary conciderably due to variety of factors but it tends to assume the average for the age group.

Efforts have been made to find out a rough and ready formula to arrive at the normal pressure figure at a given age but unfortunately no satisfactory formula has so far been found to indicate normal pressure at all ages.

All these formulae have been put forward to work out the systolic pressure only and not the diastolic.

It was once suggested that if 100 is added to the age of the individual, the figure will indicate the normal systolic pressure. However, the "age + 100" formula had to be discarded, because for the older age groups the deduced figures were often too high.

According to another formula, the normal systolic blood pressure at the age of 20 should be taken as 120 *mm Hg*, and for every 2 years of age 1 *mm Hg.* should be added to 120. This has been found satisfactory, except that it places the systolic pressure of a man aged 60 at 140 *mm Hg.* as its upper limit, a figure which is rather low for the age.

According to the third formula, 90 should be added to the age to get the normal systolic figure. This formula gives more correct figure than the age 100 formula. But it should be remembered that no formula can give the exact normal systolic figure for every individual of a particular age.

In a healthy young adult in this country belonging to age group 20-45, the systolic pressure varies between 110 and 130 *mm Hg.* of mercury.

The following table is based upon series of published figures of blood pressure estimations in the Americans.

Systolic Blood Pressure

Age	High	Average	Low
15–30 years	142	123	104
30–40 years	145	126	107
40 – 50 years	147	128	110
50–60 years	150	133	117
60 – 70 years	156	138	121

The diastolic pressure in healthy young adults is between 60 and 80 *mm Hg*. It rarely exceeds 90 and never 100 in any age group, unless there is a pathological rise of pressure.

The pulse pressure is normally about 40 to 50 *mm Hg*. But perfect health is possible with a pulse pressure as low as 30.

In women, the pressure is usually slightly lower than in man.

A variation of the systolic pressure of 20 *mm Hg.* or more is neither uncommon nor abnormal. The systolic pressure is rather unstable and is much easily affected by different factors. The diastolic pressure, on the other hand, is nearly constant – rarely varying more than 6 to 8 *mm Hg*.

While recording blood pressure, it is advisable to take at least *three* readings. The first reading is usually the highest, particularly in nervous individuals, and in those whose blood pressure has never been taken before. Usually, the third reading is much lower than the first, since by that time the patient largely, if not completely, gets over his nervousness. It is a common experience, that the blood pressure reading taken by a consultant is higher than that recorded by the family physician; a difference of 20 *mm Hg.* or more is pretty common. The reason for that is not far to seek. The patient being familiar with his own doctor does not feel as much nervous while blood pressure is being recorded, as he does feel in the presence of the consultant with whom he is not at all familiar.

The systolic reading indicates the force with which the left ventricle is contracting while the diastolic reading indicates the degree of peripheral resistance, that is, the resistance given to the flow of blood by the arterioles and capillaries. The diastolic pressure keeps the Aortic valve closed by exerting pressure upon it, and therefore, the diastolic pressure also indicates the dead-load, which the ventricle has to lift at each ventricular systole, to open up the Aortic valve and force the blood into the Aorta. Therefore, it is clear that the actual driving force for the circulation of blood is indicated neither by the systolic nor by the diastolic pressures, but by the difference between them, which is the pulse pressure.

The pressure picture is written in the following way: If the systolic pressure be 120 *mm Hg* and the diastolic be 80 *mm Hg,* the pressure picture is written as 120-80-40 or 120/80/40, the last figure indicating the pulse pressure.

Variation of Blood Pressure Under Normal Conditions

It has already been pointed out that the blood pressure of an individual is not a fixed entity. Many normal factors affect the blood pressure, causing more or less fluctuations of the pressure. These fluctuations do not indicate any disease of the heart or blood vessels.

There is frequently a DIURNAL variation of blood pressure. When one awakes normally after a good night's sleep, the blood pressure reading is the lowest for all waking hours. During the day, the blood pressure fluctuates, but it tends to rise most in the evening. During SLEEP, the blood pressure is the lowest. But in these fluctuations the systolic pressure is only affected, the diastolic pressure practically remaining constant.

POSTURE also affects blood pressure. In the recumbent position it is the lowest while when standing the systolic pressure rises by about 10 *mm Hg.;* there may be a slight rise in the diastolic pressure as well.

After a MEAL there is an appreciable rise of the systolic pressure, but not the diastolic. The bigger the meal, the greater is the rise.

In healthy individuals, EXERCISE will always cause a rise of both the systolic and the diastolic pressures ; but the systolic rise is faster and higher than the diastolic. The pulse pressure is, therefore, much increased with the purpose to enhance circulation and to meet the increased requirements of the muscles in activity. A rise of 30 to 40 *mm Hg.* in the systolic pressure is not uncommon.

Blood pressure is very greatly influenced by all EMOTIONAL STATES, like excitement, fear, anger and the like. The systolic pressure shoots up but not the diastolic, which rises but little.

All the above factors not only affect the blood pressure in the normal individual, but they also similarly affect the pressure of the hypertensives. In some patients, exercise may not cause a rise, and may even cause a fall in the pressure. This only indicates that the heart is left with little or no reserve power to rise equal to the demand made on it by exercise. Or, in other words, the heart is on its last leg.

III. Hypertension

High Blood Pressure or Hypertension

When the systolic pressure remains constantly above the upper limits of the normal for the age and sex of the individual, the condition is termed as "HYPERTENSION." It should be remembered that the systolic pressure of an individual may rise quite high in some circumstances as worry, fit of temper, etc., but so long as it is temporary it is should not be considered as hypertension. It is the continued elevation of the systolic pressure above the normal limit, which should be considered as pathological. Attention is, however, drawn to the fact that it is not at all unusual to find wide fluctuations in the systolic pressure, even in cases of chronic hypertension.

In hypertension, the diastolic pressure also rises above normal, but not to the same extent as the systolic. It also varies, but usually within narrow limits, and never as widely as the systolic. In one sense, the sustained rise of the diastolic pressure is of more important significance than that of the systolic. It has already been pointed out, that the diastolic pressure indicates the degree of peripheral resistance, which means the amount of load the heart has to lift at each beat. The higher the diastolic pressure, the greater is the load. Whenever the load is greater than normal, the condition is deemed as "Hypertension." A constant diastolic pressure of 100 *mm Hg.* or more indicates hypertension, whether or not the systolic pressure is high.

A pressure picture of 170-110-60 indicates as much hypertension as the pressure picture of 140-110-30. But there is one great difference between the above two pictures. The first picture indicates a compensated hypertension, where the heart has risen equal to the increased peripherial resistance and is maintaining an effective pulse pressure (60 *mm Hg.*) for proper circulation of blood; this picture is associated with no unpleasant symptoms. The second picture is not quite so good. The lower systolic pressure only indicates a weak heart, a heart which is not capable of pumping with enough force to maintain efficient circulation.

Of the blood is inadequate the patient may suffer from dizziness or even fainting, due to the poor supply of blood to the brain.

Therefore, only the degree of systolic pressure should not be the criterion to judge a case. The diastolic pressure, in a way, is more important than the systolic pressure. The pulse pressure is the most important factor, by which the state of the circulation of blood is gauged.

Causes of Hypertension

(a) HEREDITY – Heredity plays an importan role in its causation. If both the parents have high blood pressure, rarely the progeny escapes. If one of the parent is a hypertensive, the chance of hypertension in the children is present, but less so than in the former case.

(b) AGE – Hypertension is mostly found in people after the age of forty. But younger people do also suffer from hypertension. Many cases are seen even below the age of twenty, as also in children of about 10 years of age. The cause of hypertension may not be the same in all these people. Hypertension in children is almost always due to a chronic inflammation of the kidneys.

(c) SEX – More cases are found amongst men than in women. At or after the menopause, which is popularly known as the "change of life", women are prone to suffer from hypertension.

(d) OVER-WEIGHT AND OBESITY – More cases of hypertension are found in the over-weight and obese individuals, than in thin and under-weight people. They are often of low stature with stumpy limbs and short neck.

(e) INTEMPERANCE IN DRINK AND OVER-INDULGENCE IN FOOD – There is no evidence to support, that moderate use of alcohol has any causative relation to blood pressure. But over-indulgence in alcohol may be a contributory factor, either by its poisonous effect, or by its capacity to make the drinker obese and stout.

Meat-eaters are not more prone to blood pressure than the vegetarians. It is the quantity of food that matters. Over-indulgence in rich food, particularly when prolonged for years, will lead to stoutness and increased pressure.

All sorts of vicious dissipations are likely to lead to this trouble.

(f) MENTAL STATES – People, who are unfortunately so placed in life as to suffer from continual anxiety or worry for many years, tend to become chronic hypertensives. A continued and sustained rise of blood pressure for a long stretch of time, caused by such mental factor may ultimately become a permanent disease.

(g) PERSONALITY – A type of high blood pressure known as "Essential Hypertension" is often associated with a distinctive personality type. The patients are usually hyper-active individuals, with great exuberance of mental and physical energy. They are temperamentally restless and always look for work. They are usually sensitive and short-tempered. Some of them appear to be at the very *pick* of health.

How the Heart and Blood Vessels are Affected

From pathologic point, the CEREBRAL ARTERIES come next to CORONARY VESSLES and the AORTA in their susceptibility to Atherosclerosis.

In Essential Hypertension, the most usual points of attack are, the HEART, the EYES, the BRAIN and the KIDNEYS.

There are *three* types of changes seen in blood vessels:-

(a) The ARTERIOLES are the first to be affected –

fatty hyaline changes and the homogeneous swelling of the walls occur.

(b) In the MEDIUM ARTERIES – Hypertrophy and internal thickening occur.

(c) In the LARGE ARTERIES – Atheromatous degeneration of the intima occur.

These arteriolar changes tend to increase the peripheral resistance, resulting in acceleration of arteriosclerotic and atheromatous changes in larger vessels, including the Aorta, the Coronaries and the Cerebral ones.

Coronary Vessels

The strain on the left vertricle and the state of coronary circulation determine the cardiac output in normal cases.

The increased peripheral resistance increases the work of the left ventricle resulting in its ultimate concentric hypertrophy to compensate for the extra load imposed.

This left ventricular hypertrophy increases the muscle mass, but with it, the increase in coronary vascular bed is not commensurated upon, hence resulting in myocardial Ischemia and failure.

Another factor to be taken into consideration along with it, is the development of Coronary arteriosclerosis which aggravates myocardial ischemia leading to Myocardial infarction.

The renal insufficiency as the sequelea to myocardial failure leads to retention of sodium and water and hence agreeably invites cardiac failure.

Pulse

The more severe the hypertension, the smaller is that amplitude of the pulse.

The large amplitude, *i. e.,* the full, bounding pulse shows systolic hypertension (Atherosclerosis) and not diastolic.

Common Pathology

In every case of hypertension there is an increase in the peripheral resistance. This increased peripheral resistance may also be increased due to the interference with capillary circulation in the kidneys, or due to the inflammation of these organs.

Usually the initial cause of chronic hypertension is the spasm of the arterioles throughout the body. If the spasm would continue for months and years, there will be eventual organic change in the arteriolar walls, tending to make them rigid and thick, and thus, causing the narrowing of the passages through them. As long as the organic change of the arteriolar walls has not occurred, the blood pressure could be restored to normal, if the cause of the vasospasm could be obviated. Even with advanced organic changes in the arterioles, there is some degree of vasospasm present, which, of course, is of no moment.

By a simple test, which is safely applicable to all cases except those who are very seriously ill, one can determine which of the two factors–*spasm* or *organic change*–is dominating in a hypertensive.

Inhalation of a drug called "*Amyl nitrite*" causes a wide-spread vaso-dilatation, though only for a short while. Or, in other words, "*Amyl nitrite*" removes the spasm of the arterioles. By observing the effect of "*Amyl nitrite*" inhalation, on both the systolic and diastolic pressures, it can be concluded as to how much part the spasm or organic change of the arterioles plays in a case of hypertension.

Procedure of the Test

(a) Take the blood pressure reading and note it down.

(b) Maintain sufficient pressure in the armlet, so that the click of the first phase remains audible.

(c) Let the patient inhale a capsule of *"Amyl nitrite"*, crushed in a bit of cotton wool.

(d) If spasm be present, it will soon pass off by the action of the drug, and the blood pressure will fall. Therefore, within a few minutes of inhalation, the click will no longer be heard.

(e) Release the pressure in the armlet by means of the escape-valve, and locate the lowest systolic and diastolic pressures.

(f) The degree of blood pressure drop indicates the intensity of the vascular spasm in the patient.

It is not unusual to find a pulse pressure of 100 *mm Hg.* to drop to 40 to 50 *mm Hg.* after *"Amyl nitrite"* inhalation. Any physician in active practice might have observed a pressure picture of 240-130-110 changing to 130-78-52 by this test, indicating that the rise of peripheral resistance in this case was on account of arteriolar spasm.

If, on the other hand, the hypertensive would show little or no drop in the blood pressure by this test, it only proves that spasm plays very little or no part in this case, and that advanced organic change has occurred in the arterioles, which have become incapable of dilatation.

By means of the above test we can make out the underlying cause of increased peripheral resistance. In some cases the absorption of toxin from acute or chronic foci of infection seems to be responsible for spasm. Since the removal of such foci has restored the blood pressure to normal in some patients though not in all, showing focal sepsis. Cases are on record, in whom the draining of an abscess, removal of a tooth with an apical collection of pus, taking out of a diseased gall-bladder or appendix have brought the pressure down to normal.

In toxemias of pregnancy – including Eclampsia, the toxin is supposed to be responsible for the spasm of the arterioles, as well as for the inflammation of the kidneys. With the evacuation of the uterus the source of toxin is removed, and, in consequence, the blood pressure comes down to normal in a few weeks in the large majority of cases.

Blood pressure may also rise due to the disorder or imbalance of the glands of internal secretion which influence the arterioles. Raised blood pressure is seen in cases of Exophthalmic goitre, in Pituitary tumors, and sometimes after Menopause.

A rise of blood pressure is also observed in cases of acute inflammation of the kidneys, which is known as

"Acute glomerulo-nephritis" –a condition which is often associated with edema, scanty urine or suppression of urine, albuminuria, hematuria and fever. If the Acute nephritis completely clears up, the blood pressure returns to normal and continues to remain so. But sometimes the acute inflammation of the kidneys subsides only to exist in a chronic form.

The arteriolar conditions can be seen directly through the eyes, hence Retinoscopy serves a very useful means as a diagnostic agent in hypertensive cases. Retinal findings serve as reliable index to the serverity of the condition.

Ophthalmic examination may reveal :—

(a) Thickening of the arterioles,

(b) Exudates,

(c) Small punctiform hemorrhages,

(d) Thrombosis,

(e) Papilledema,

Regarding arterial thickenings Paul wood mentions:

(a) Increased tortuousness of the blood-vessels in the retina.

(b) Notching or kinking of veins at arterio-venous crossings.

(c) Irregular narrowing of the arteries.

(d) White fringes or lines along, denoting thickening of the arterial walls.

(e) The silver-wire artery owing to complete occlusion of its lumen.

In hypertensions, the retinal arteries appear narrower than the veins along with them. Paul wood says that this is the most marked and important sign in essential hypertension.

Chronic Hypertension

Chronic hypertension, with which we are chiefly concerned, falls under the following heads :–

(a) Hypertension due to Chronic nephritis.

(b) Essential hypertension–
   • benign   • malignant.

(c) Climacteric hypertension, or Hypertension of Menopause.

Hypertension Due to Chronic nephritis

History

A history of previous fever with edema, scanty urine, albuminuria, hematuria etc., makes the diagnosis easy, by drawing our attention to the kidneys. In all probability, the acute inflammation of the kidneys never completely cleared up, put continued in existence because the previous Acute nephritis might have been so mild as not present the typical picture, as mentioned above. More often a history of recurrent attacks of Tonsillitis, sore-throat, easy susceptibility to cold, repeated attacks of Flue – or in short–a history of previous trouble of the upper respiratory passages is available. These upper respiratory infections are very prone to affect the kidneys, and therefore, the history of such infection should draw our attention to them.

Blood Pressure

In Chronic nephritis, the blood pressure is usually not excessively high. A systolic pressure between 160 and 180 and a diastolic pressure between 100 and 120 are common observations. But exceptions are sometimes found, with higher pressure figures.

The Urine

On enquiry, the patient would often say, that there is nothing wrong with his urine. On a careful questioning, he will say that he repeatedly passes large quantity of urine "as clear as water." This brings out two important points–

one, *an increase in the total volume of urine,* and the other, *want of concentration of urine,* that is, *low specific gravity,*

The increase of total volume and the constant low specific gravity of the urine indicate poor function of the kidneys. When these organs function properly a large quantity of water will produce thin watery urine, while, when the fluid intake is low, the urine will be concentrated (or high specific gravity) and high-coloured. This failure in the ability of the kidneys to concentrate urine will produce a large volume of urine, which should be got rid of by frequency urination (Polyuria) by day as well as by night (Nocturia). The loss of large quantity of water from the body will cause frequent thirst (Polydipsia), which is nothing but the cry of nature for restoration of the fluids usually and continuously lost in the urine.

Examination of the urine will usually reveal a trace of albumin, though in certain cases the albumin reaction may be quite marked. All varieties of casts may be met with. Presence of a few red blood corpuscles and a few pus cells may also be found.

But the most reliable and constant findings are the increase in the total volume and low specific gravity of all specimens of urine, showing a trace of albumin.

With the progressive impairment of the functional capacity of the kidneys, which are the most important organs of elimination of waste products from the blood, there will be progressive retention of these products in the blood. This retention will ultimately lead to Uremia, a fatal complication.

Edema or Swelling

In most cases the edema is slight and fleeting. Slight puffiness of the face and particularly of eye-lids in the morning may be noticed, which usually passes off during the day. Occasionally, the edema may be very marked.

Essential Hypertension

Selection of Cases

During hypertensive therapy, the physician often cuts a sorry figure when he discovers after a time that he was treating a patient for Essential hypertension, while it had been due to renal, endocrine or some other cause and it would be even unforgivable if there were no hypertension existing at all.

So, the determination of Basal blood pressure is important. Not one, but several readings should be taken when the patient is fully relaxed both in mind and body.

In doubtful cases, allow seven days complete rest in bed even with adequate sedation.

A diastolic pressure conistently above 90 *mm. Hg.* should arouse suspicion.

Two exceptions may however be mentioned here; In very obese and in arteriosclerotic patients, the diastolic pressure above 100 *mm. Hg.* might be considered as normal.

The diagnosis of Essential hypertension must necessarily be made after excluding renal, endocrine, vascular and neurological causes.

A case of Essential hypertension can be BENIGN or MALIGNANT, according to the functional condition of the kidneys. As a matter of fact, the benign and the malignant hypertensions are not two different diseases, but they are two stages of the same and progressive pathological process. When the Hypertension is associated with normal kidney function, it is BENIGN, whereas association with deranged kidney functions would make the very same case MALIGNANT.

History

Essential hypertension will often reveal the history of hypertension in one or both the parents. But ther are many cases, which would furnish no such history. The patient usually gives the personal history of perfect health in the past, and may even boast that he never had a doctor in his life. He usualy looks healthy and robust, with a glow of health on his face. His hypertension is often discovered, for the first time, not on account of any related symptoms, but accidentally—by a chance of examination of his bood pressure, as for taking out a life insurance policy. Essential hypertension is commonly found in the third to the fifth decade of life.

Blood Pressure

The blood pressure is often exceedingly high. It is not unusual to get the systolic reading of 200 *mm Hg.* or more. The diastolic is about 130 *mm Hg.* But it should be borne in mind that lesser readings do not negative the diagnosis.

The Urine

In the benign stage, there is nothing wrong with functions of the kidneys. The quantity and the quality of urine is normal, and its specific gravity changes according to the quantity of fluid in-take. The concentrating power of the kidneys is manifest in low fluid intake, by the secretion of urine of high colour and high specific gravity. There is no polyuria, nocturia or polydipsia. Examination of urine gives normal analytical result, though occasionally a trace of albumin may be found. Inhalation of *"Amyl nitrite"* brings down the systolic and diastolic pressures to normal, or very near normal.

When the case gradually drifts towards the malignant side, the kidney functions progressively deteriorate. Polyuria, nocturia, polydipsia, and constantly low specific gravity of the urine are found. Albuminuria makes its appearance. *"Amyl nitrite"* does not bring down the pressure as low as formerly.

Climacteric Hypertension

It is very much like the Essential hypertension of the benign type. The rise of pressure is mainly due to vascular spasm, as could be proved by *"Amyl nitrite"* inhalation. The patient is above forty-five years of age, and is usually stout, over-weighed, under-sized, and mother of many children. Such patients have remarkable tolerance for high blood pressure, and do not usually suffer from any or much discomfort, even when the pressure is very high.

Significance of the Symptoms in Hypertensions

Although the signs, *i.e.,* the physical findings in a patient during the physician's examination of his patients are indispensible, yet the symptoms recorded are more important than the signs, especially in some diseases at least, hence arises the question of very careful minute history-taking.

In hypertension, an untreated patient may remain asymptomatic for even 10 to 12 years, although, once he be made aware of it, he is sure to complain headache, giddiness, fatigue, nervousness, palpitation and loss of concentration.

Although these may be the outcome of anxiety, yet put together they all point towards complications arising out of hypertension.

Leishman rightly asserts, "If a man is fated to die from hypertension, he will do so from Heart failure, Uremia, Cardiac infraction or Stroke."

Paul Wood explains the occurence of such symptoms to be due to selective vaso-constriction *i.e.,* more vaso-constriction in the brain area, than in the skin area.

Symptoms of Hypertension

Symptoms do not appear as soon as the pressure tends to rise. As a matter of fact, active and vigorous mental and bodily health is possible with hypertension. For some years, perhaps, there has been a gradual increase of the pressure, of which the patient has not been aware. Often patients have no complaints before a physician tells them about their heightened blood pressure.

When, however, the pressure reaches the limit of the patient's tolerance, symptoms begin to appear. Commonly, the nervous symptoms appear first, which are noticed either by the patient himself, or by his friends and relations. Irritability of temper, nervousness, change of dispostion, inability to concentrate the mind, throbbing headache, insomnia and giddiness are some of the common initial symptoms. Rapid failure of vision, or even sudden blindness due to retinal hemorrhage, may be the first symptom to attract attention to the blood pressure.

With the deterioration of the function of the kidneys, the urinary symptoms appear and puffiness, more or less, under the eyes is noticed in the morning.

When the heart is embarrassed by the increased load of peripheral resistance, breathlessness on slight exertion and cough make their appearance. Soon after edema of the ankles starts, which is particularly marked in the evening after the day's work, but may disappear in the morning after a good night's rest. Precordial distress and even anginal pain, may be experienced. When heart failure becomes very marked, there is great dyspnea, even at rest, cough with bloody expectoration, anasarca and scanty high-coloured urine.

Hemorrhage in and from different parts of the body is met with in cases of hypertension. Bleeding from nose and gums is common, and is deemed beneficial since such bleeding may be considered as a safety-valve action. Bleeding in the lungs is also met with, which reveals itself as haemoptysis of different intensity. Hemorrhage in the brain, known as "Apoplexy", is a very serious condition, which kills the patient outright, or leaves him to the miserable existence of a paralytic; only occasionally a complete or almost complete recovery is seen.

The Blood Pressure Regime

Most modern scientists are of opinion that this is a disease where over-treatment kills more than under-treatment.

High blood pressure and hypertensive diseases are not the same things.

Blood pressure must of necessity be variable, adapting itself to environments. Excitement, fear, anger, exertion, etc., all mental upheavals, influence the blood pressure. Many carry on a long healthy life in spite of all the ups and downs. Some requiring simple reassurances from a personality, others carry on well with simple managment of diet control and a change in the tempo of life, a few requiring only mild hypotensive drugs occasionally.

However, the careful physician must never lose sight of the etiology—the primary disease—bringing on this hypertension in its trail

The hypertensive should be made to understand, that he will have to live a very well-regulated and methodical life, if he wants to prolong it without suffering. It is far better to tell the patient frankly that his blood pressure would remain above normal, in stead of leading him into false hopes. But at the same time, it must be explained that elevated pressure is compatible with good health, unless it is too much elevated. As a matter of fact, an elevated pressure is essential for his life, as it determines adequate circulation of blood through the body. But at the same time he must be made to understand that he should take precaution, so that his blood pressure does not shoot up and bring about an accident.

REST

The value of rest, both physical and mental, in the management of high blood pressure is very considerable. A hypertensive should live as quiet a life as practicable, and should avoid all sorts of mental irritation, worry and bother. He should by no means get into avoidable controversy, debate and the like. He should maintain a cool temper, and never lose it, He should undertake no sudden exertion, and never hurry. Straining at stool should be scrupulously avoided. A good bit of rest and sleep every day should be ensured. Sometimes much benefit occurs from keeping the patient in bed for a day or so. Moderate and regulated exercise should not be discouraged. Walking is an excellent form of exercise. Quiet cycling, golf, horse-riding, swedish exercises and slow breathing exercises may be allowed in some cases. "The *cardinal rule*", as said by Price, "in all cases should be that exercise should not be carried to the point of increased frequency of pulse and respiration, or indication of cardiac distress." An hour's rest after a meal should be done.

DIET

The nature of diet should depend on the type of the case under consideration. However, too drastic regulation of diet is not often required; it only tends to make the patient miserable. But in every case of hypertension, one should see that the meals are neither large, nor rich. Spicy foods and fats should be avoided. Meat should either be omitted from the dietary, or allowed only once a week, in a very small quantity. Meat extractives, like soup and gravy, are better forbidden. Milk and white meat, like chicken or fish, may be safely allowed. Carbohydrates, fresh vegetables and fruits have no contraindication, unless the patient is obeise where the carbohydrate should be reduced. Tea is allowed in moderation, but it is better to avoid coffee. Alcohol is better left alone altogether. Food should be taken at regular hours and should be eaten slowly and thoroughly masticated. Addition of table salt at meals is better avoided, as well as large drinks of water.

In stout hypertensives, and particularly in those with very high blood pressure, an initial day of fast followed by a few days of fruit and milk diet, has been found useful. Good results have been found in patients, who observe two days of fasting in the month. Reduction of weight in obese individuals by under-dieting is beneficial.

Indulgence in tobacco is either completely stopped, or, if that is not possible, is allowed only in small quantity.

In dictaries of the obese, 1500 calories will be up to the mark.

In normal cases, drinking of salt-water brings in hypertension, so, it is advised that even a-symptomatic hypertensives should exercise a check on *sodium* intake, *i.e.,* below 500 grms. per day.

But here GILCHRIST draws our attention to the "salt depletion syndrome and points his warning finger to the characteristic symptoms following salt restriction, nausea vomiting, weakness and collapse.

He, however, recommends a little addition of salt to the dietary after 2 to 3 weeks restriction.

Low *sodium* diet is contra-indicated in cases where the specific gravity of urine is below 1015, according to some observers.

BOWELS

Steps should be taken that the bowels move satisfactorily and regularly. Such movement is of greater value than an occasional severe purge. Good wash of the bowels twice a month has been found to help in some cases. Attempts should first be made to regulate bowels by dietetic measures, before taking recourse to drugs.

BATH

Cold bath should be avoided, as it tends to rise blood pressure. Tepid or warm bath is advocated. Hot bath, once or twice a week, sometimes helps.

THERAPY

In treating a case of hypertension, GILCHRIST warns the treating physician never to tell his patient that his disease was becoming worse and drugs were proving valueless.

FISHBERG's suggestion on this point is that every effort must be made to help a hypertensive patient with his mental or emotional troubles.

The patient should certainly need advice on ways of his life, habits and occupation. The patient should be well-advised to get his ways of life well-adapted to his blood pressure.

A short rest after mid-day meal, long hours of sleep in the night, a quiet retired week-end rest, annual holiday sojourn and avoidance of all bustles and irritative tussles should strictly be enjoined.

The patient should be advised to live the life of a Hindu widow cultivating philosophical temperament, temperate habits and theistic attitude.

Mental relaxation is as essential as physical relaxation, and sound sleep relieves much strain on the vascular system even if it be for a few hours.

Caution in Treating Cases of Hypertension

In treating cases of hypertension, the physician should keep in mind that the severity of cases depend not on the blood pressure level, but on the condition of the arterioles.

Bad prognosis in hypertension lies in the complications.

RENAL, CEREBRAL and CARDIAC.

The treatment must go on keeping a close watch

on :—

(a) Condition of arterioles revealed in retinoscopy,

(b) Efficiency in the working of the cardiac machinery,

(c) Renal disfunction.

Hypertensive Therapy

Asympotomatic hypertension requires no treatment, this was the definite opinion of the past observers, but in view of the new researches, some change in their attitude has been brought to bear upon this subject.

(a) Firstly, hypertension leads to hypertensive diseases.

(b) Unrelieved high diastolic pressure brings in malignant hypertension.

(c) There is no certainty that the asymptomatic stage will not end in a symptomatic condition.

MAYER says, "There is no need to treat cases whose diastolic pressure is not above 100 *mm Hg.* and in cases with diastolic pressure above 100 but below 110 *mm. Hg,* treat only the progressive cases or them with complications."

FISHBERG even asserts, "hypertensives would have been more fortunate if hypertensions had not been discovered."

But most modern investigators are of opinion that it would be wise to lower the blood presure even in the early stage of hypertension. They even contend that in cases of hypertensions having diastolic pressure above 120*mm Hg.* symptoms are bound to appear within two to three years, if left untreated, especially in men.

IV. Hypotension

Hypotension or Low Blood Pressure

In dealing with the disorders of blood pressure the question of hypotension cannot be ignored with impunity. True it is, that hypertension has engaged the attention of the profession infinitely more than hypotension. The reason for this lies in the fact, that the former is more often associated with grave danger and consequence, while the latter is not half so dangerous to life provided there is no serious associated conditions.

Now the question arises as to what systolic pressure should be considered as sub-normal. An individual having as low a systolic pressure as 100 *mm. Hg.* may enjoy perfect health. There is no reason why he should not do so, provided his pulse pressure remains over 30 *mm. Hg.* However, in some persons with such a low pressure, symptoms like headache, vertigo, muscular fatigue, mental lassitude, constipation due to reduced intestinal tone, etc., are produced. These symptoms need attention, since they indicate a pathological state.

Definition

It is indeed diffcult to furnish a dogmatic definition of hypotnsion. But as a rough working rule, a systolic pressure between 80—100 *mm. Hg.* should be considered to indicate hypotension. However, it should be borne in mind, that the pressure may be much above 100 and yet below for an individual.

It has already been pointed out that normal pressure value is not the same in all individuals of the same age group, though the variation usually lies within certain limits. So long as the normal pulse pressure is maintained and no symptoms are produced, the blood pressure should be considered as normal and not low, even though the readings do not conform to those of the age group, to which the individual may belong. Only when a low reading is associated with characteristic symptoms, the condition should be deemed as hypotension.

Primary and Secondary Hypotension

Primary Hypotension

Primay hypotension is a condition for which no cause could be assigned. Probably the factors responsible for low pressure are conveyed to the family by heredity. There are families, whose members habitually carry hereditary or famillial hypotension is not quite so common.

Secondary Hypotension

Secondary hypotension is commoner. The cases are numerous, and they are always the results of some PRIMARY malady. The causes of secondary hypotension may be classified as follows : –

(a) **Acute Infections** : Excepting cerebro-spinal meningitis, all acute infective diseases cause a fall in the blood pressure.

(b) **Chronic Wasting Diseases** : Diabetes, Tuberculosis and malnutrition from whatever cause.

(c) **Endocrine Disease** : Addison's disease.

(d) **Fluid Loss from the Body** : Hemorrhage, profuse diarrheoa, Cholera etc.

(e) **Cardio-vascular Diseases** : Dilatation of the heart, Myocarditis, Mitral stenosis, Arteriosclerosis (in some cases) and failing heart before death.

(f) **Nervous Diseases** : Neuroasthenia, after epileptic fits and after lumbar puncture, exhaustion, anaphylactic and surgical shocks.

(g) **Blood Dyscrasias** : Anemia, primary or secondary, Leukemia, and Polycythemia with Splenomegaly.

(h) **Intoxications** : Chloroform and tobacco (chronic).

Disadvantages of Hypotension

People who suffer from hypotension are unable to carry on with their normal pursuits in life with vigour and, in bad cases, may not be able to live comfortably even at home. Any change of posture, particularly when assuming the upright position from the recumbent position – causes a fall in the pulse pressure, due to the low vascular tone, especially in the splanchnic vessels. The fall causes giddiness, and may even cause fainting, due to a temporary poverty of blood in the brain.

Hypotension is also an important factor in the production of cerebral as well as coronary thrombosis. In diseased arteries (Arteriosclerosis) a slow blood stream, which is inevitable with hypotension, is a contributory cause for intravascular clotting. As a matter of fact, most cases of coronary and cerebral thrombosis come across in people, who have been sufferingfrom Arteriosclerosis with hypotension

Finally, a hypotensive has a poor resistance to infection, which, when contracred, would worsen the case by a further reduction of pressure.

Need for Energitic Hypotension

It will be well to remember that Energetic hypotensive therapy will be needed in all cases, (a) manifesting hypertensive retinopathy, (b) without Retinopathy, but having had transient cerebro-vascular episodes, left ventricular failure or Angina pectoris and (c) Diastolic hypertension above 120 *mm Hg.*, associated with severe headache.

Management of Hypotension

It is obvious that the treatment of SECONDARY HYPOTENSION centres round the treatment of the *primary* cause. If the *primary* cause is amenable to treatment, the associated hypotension will tend to disappear.

PRIMARY HYPOTENSION, when not attended with any symptom, need not be bothered with at all. Only those cases, which are associated with symptoms as already mentioned, should be attended to. Though in many cases, it is almost impossible to cause any great rise of the pressure, yet observation shows that, in a hypotensive, a slight increase in tension is attended with subjective improvement, which is out of all proportion to the increase in pressure. In the management of these cases, *general hygienic measures* are as important as remedial drugs.

Contra-indications for Energetic Hypotension Therapy

(a) Patients above 60 years having arteriosclerotic degeneration where the result of such therapy would be harmful.

(b) Patients having evidences of Coronary insufficiency.

(c) Patients with marked impairment of renal function.

(d) Very mild hypertension cases.

General Management

(a) Attend to the *hygiene* of the mouth, teeth and throat, and correct *constipation* which is frequent, by dietetic means or by weak natural laxatives. Strong purgatives must not be given.

(b) Correct *under-nutrition* by appetising, with wholesome and vitaminous food; but do not allow rich or heavy meal, which might upset the digestion. Meat soup or extractives should be included in the dietary.

(c) *Rest* is an important factor. Instruct to retire early to bed and rise early, if possible. The patient should be advised to make the process of getting up from bed a slow and gradual process, and not jumpy, by any chance. Rest for an hour in bed should also be enjoined after each meal.

(d) *Massage* and *exercise* should be prescribed. General massage has a stimulating effect. An oil massage before bath is helpful. Bodily exercise should be prescribed, in accordance with the condition and the age of the patient. If he is restricted to bed, he should be given a few breathing exercises, which will stimulate the circulation of blood.

This effect could be enhanced by a simple abdominal exercise as follows : Ask the patient to draw in the anterior abdominal wall and hold it on as long as possible, at intervals of 2 to 5 minutes for 10 to 15 times, morning and evening.

Patients, who are not so ill, should take towel or free hand exercises, particulary the abdominal ones. They should, however, be *warned* not to over-step their safe limits, and be exhausted and breathless.

(e) *Hydrotherapy :*

- Hot and cold *shower* bath. This is the *best* when available. After the exercise, the patient stands under a shower of warm water, which gradually and slowly changes into hot. The hot shower is suddenly turned off, and a shower of ordinary cold water is started, which is gradually and slowly changed into as cold as could be well-borne. Turn off the shower and treat as below.

- Hot and cold *sponge* bath. Give a hot sponging to the whole body, except the head. Then quickly sponge with cold fresh or salt water. Next pour a bucket of cold water on the back and spine an treat as below.

After the bath, follow immediately by a brisk rubbing with a coarse towel, to produce redness of the skin. Dry and cover him up with blankets or sheets. Keep him in recumbent position for half an hour.

Intoxication : Stop all excessive indulgence in tobacco, alcohol, tea and coffee. Correct all detrimental habits, which are too many to enumerate individually.

On Prognosis Hypertension as Furnished by Gilchrist

	Mild Cases	Moderately	Very severe cases
1. Symptoms	Nil or Slight Morning Headache and Vertigo	Moderate Frequent Headaches, Fatigue, Dyspnoea and Nocturia	Severe Intense Headache, Weakness, Loss of weight, Dyspnea and Confusion
2. Blood Pressure	150 to 200 100 to 120	180 to 280 110 to 140	240 to 300 130 to 180
3. Retina	Minimal Arterial narrowing to definite sclerosis	Definite Sclerosis with Exudates, Star figures, Cotton wool patches or Hemorrhages, Definite Retinitis	Papilledema with advanced Retinitis with Star figures. Cotton wool Patches or Hemorrhages
4. Renal Functions	Normal to Satisfactory Faint trace of Albumen occasional	Impaired Albumen with Casts and RBC	Impaired Albumen with Casts and RBC Progressively dateriorating
5. Mortality Rates	20% to 25%	75%	

V. Repertory on Blood Pressure

MIND

ABRUPT – N a t - m . Tarent.

ABSENT-MINDED — Agn. Alum. **APIS.** Arn. **Aur. Bar-c. Calad. CANN-I. CAUST. Cham.** Dulc. Graph. **Hell.** Hep. Ign. Kali-br. **Kali-c. Kali-p.** Lac-c. **LACH. Lyc.** Mag-c. Merc. **Mez.** Mosch. **NAT-M. Nux-m. Nux-v.** Op. Petr. **Ph-ac.** Phos. **PLAT.** Plb. **Puls.** Rhus-t. **SEP.** Sil. Sulph. Thuj. **VERAT.** Zinc.

ANGER—Acon. **ANAC. Ars. BELL. BRY. CHAM.** Hep. **Hyos.** Ign. **Kali-c.** kali-s. **LYC. Merc. Mosch. NAT-M. NIT-AC. NUX-V. Petr.** Psor. **Sep. STAPH. Stram.** Tarent. Verat.

ANGUISH—**ACON.** Apis. Arg-n. Arn. **Ars. Aur. BELL.** Bism. **Calc. Cann-I. CAUST.** Coff. **Crot-h.** Cupr.

Dig. Hep. Hyos. Mag-c. Naja Nat-c. **Phos. PLAT.** Psor. Puls. Sep. Tarent. Verat.

ANXIETY—ACON. Ambr. Anac. Ant-t. **ARG-N.** Asar. Bar-c. **BELL. BISM. BOR.** Bry. Calc. Camph. Cann-I. **Carb-s. CAUST.** Cocc. **Con.** Ferr. **Gels.** Graph. **Iod. KALI-C. Kali-p.** Kali-s. **LYC.** Mez. Nat-a. **NIT-AC.** Nux-v. **Petr.** Phos-ac. Psor. **PULS.** Sep. Sil. Stram. Tab. Thuj. Zinc.

APHASIA — **ARS.** BRY. Calc. Cina. Coloc. **Lyc.** Nat-c. **Puls.** Sep.

BUSINESS, AVERSE TO — Agar. Anac. Ars. **Brom.** Cimi. **Con.** Graph. Kali-bi. Kali-br. Kali-c **Lach.** Mag-s. **PHOS-AC.** Phyt. **Puls. Sep.** Sulph.

CHILOISH BEHAVI-OUR — Anac. **Apis. BAR-C.** Bar-m. Carb-an. Carb-s. **CIC.**

Croc. Ign. Kali-br. **Nux-m.** Puls. Seneg. **Stram.** Viol-o.

COMPANY; AVERSION TO—Aloe Ambr. **ANAC. Aur. BAR-C.** Bell. **Bry.** Cact. Calc-p. **Carb-an.** Carb-v **CHAM.** Cupr. Ferr. **GELS.** Hell. Hep. **IGN.** Iod. Kali-br. Kali-c. Lac-d. Lach. **LYC.** Nat-c. **NAT-M. NUX-V. Phos.** pic-ac. **Plat. Puls. Sel. Sep.** Stann. **Sulph.** Thuj. Verat.

CONCENTRATION, DIFFICULT—Ambr. **ANAC.** Apis. **BAR-C. Cann-I.** Carb-an. **Carb-s. CARB-V. CAUST.** Cocc. Con.Dulc. Gels. **Graph.** Hydr. **Hyos.** Kali-br. Kali-c. Kali-p. Lac-c. **LACH. LYC.** Mag-m. Med. Merc. Mez. **Nat-a.** Nat-c. **Nat-m.** Nit-ac. **NUX-M. NUX-V.** Op. **PHOS-AC. PHOS.** Pic-ac. Plat. Puls. Rhus-t. **Sel. SEP. SIL.** Spong. Stram. Sulph. Ter. Thuj. Verat. Viol-o. Zinc.

CONFUTION OF MIND—**Anac.** Ant-t. Arg-n. Ars. **Aur.** Bapt. **BELL.** Bor. **Bry.**

CALC. Caps. **CARB-V.** Chin. Coff. Crot-h, Dios. **Ferr. Gels. GLON.** Graph. Hyos. **LACH.** Lyc. Mag-c. **MERC.** Mez. **Mosch.** Nat-c. **NAT-M.** Nit-ac. **Nux-m. Nux-v. Onos. OP. Petr.** Phos-ac. **Phos.** Plb. Puls. **Rhus-t.** Sabad. Seneg. **SEP.** Staph. **Stram. Stry.** Sulph. Syph. Valer. **Zinc.**

CONSOLATION AGG. – Arn. **Ars. Bell.** Cact. Calc-p. **Cham.** Hell. **Ign.** Kali-c. Lil-t. **Lyc. NAT**-m. Nit-ac. Nux-v. **Plat. SEP. SIL.** Staph. Tarent.

CONSOLATION AMEL. –**PULS.**

CONTEMPTUOUS - Ars. Canth. **Cham.** Chin. **CIC.** Hyos. Ign. Lach. **Lyc.** Nat-m. **Nit-ac. PLAT.** Sil.

CONTRADICT, DISPOSITION TO—Anac. **Aur.** Canth. **Caust.** Ferr. **HEP.** Hyos. **Ign.** Lach. **Lyc.** Merc. Nat-c. Nit-AC. **Nux-v.** Olnd.Ruta

CONTRADICTION, IS INTOLERANT OF–Aloe.

Anac. **Aur. Bry.** Cocc. Ferr. Helon. **IGN. LYC.** Merc. Nat-c. **NUX-V.** Op. Petr. **Sep.** Sil. Stram.

CURSING—Aloe. **ANAC.** Ars. **Bell.** Cann-s. **Canth. Hyos.** Lac-c. **Lil-t. Lyc.** Nat-m. **NIT-AC. Nux-v.** Op. Plb. Puls. **Stram.** Tub. **Verat.**

DELUSIONS—Ambr. **ARG-N. Ars.** Aur. Bapt. **BELL.** Calc. **CANN-I. Cann-s.** Caust. **Cocc.** Coff. **GLON.** Hell. **HYOS.** Ign. Kali-br. **LACH.** Lyc.Lyss. Merc. **Nit-ac.** Op. **Petr. Phos-ac.** Phos. Psor. Puls. Rhus-t. **SABAD.** Sec. Sil. **STRAM. Sulph. Zinc.**

FORGETFUL—AMBR. **Anac.** Arg-n. Aur. **BAR-C.**Calc.Carb-s. Colch. Kali-br. **KALI-P.** Lach. **LYC.** Merc. **Nat-m.** Nux-v **Petr. PHOS-AC. PHOS. Plat.** Ruta **Selen.** Sep. **Sulph.** Thuj. Tub. Verat. **Zinc.**

FRIGHTENED EASILY —Arg-n. **ARS. Bar-c.** Bell. **BOR.** Bry. Calc. Carb-an. **Caust. GRAPH.** Hyos. **Ign. Kali-c.**

kali-p. **LYC. Merc. Nat-a. NAT-C. Nat-m.** Nux-v. **OP.** Petr. Phos. **PULS. STRAM.** Sulph. Ther. Verat.

HURRY—Apis. **ARG-N.ARS.** Bar-c. Bell. Camph. Carb-s. Coff. Crot-c. Graph. **Hep.** Hyos. Ign. kali-c. **kali-p. Lach. LIL-T. MED. MERC.** Mosch. Nat-c. **NAT-M. Nux-V.** Phos-ac. **Phos.** Puls. Stram. **SULPH, Sulph-ac. Tarent.** Thuj. Verat.

IMBECILITY—Aloe. **AMBR.** Am-c. **ANAC.** Arg-n. Ars. Aur. **BAR-C. Bar-m. Bell. BUFO. Carb-s.** Caust. Cocc. **CON.** Dios. **Hyos.** Ign. Kali-p. Lac-c. **Lyc.** Merc. **Nux-m. Nux-v. Op. Phos-ac. Sil.** Staph. **STRAM. Sulph.** Ther. **Verat.** Verb, Zinc.

INDOLENCE—Aur. **CALC. Carb-s. Chel. CHIN.** Cycl. **GRAPH.** Hep. Ign. Iod. Kali-c. Lac-c. **LACH.** Mez. **NAT-M. NIT-AC. Nux-v.** Phos-ac. Phos. **Pic-ac.** Psor. **Puls. SEP.** Stann. **SULPH.** Ther. Thuj. zinc.

LOQUACITY—Arg-m. Aur. BELL. Camph. Cann-I. Cimi. Croc. Crot-c. Cupr. Ferr-p. Gels. HYOS. Kali-br. LACH. Lachn. Mur-ac. Nat-c. Nux-v. OP. Phos. Plb. Podo. Pyrog. Selen. STRAM. Sulph. Thea. Thuj. Verat.

MILDNESS —Arn. Ars. Ars-i. BOR. Cact. Calad. Calc. Cann-I. Caust. Cocc. Croc. Cupr. Hell. Ign. Indg. Kali-c. Lil-t. Lyc. Mosch. Nit-ac. NAT-M. OP. Phos-ac. Phos. Plb. PULS. Rhus-t. Sep. SIL. Spong. Stann. Stram. Sulph. Thuj. Verat. Zinc.

MISTAKES LOCALI- TIES— Bell. Cann-I. Cic. GLON. Hura. Lach. Merc. Nat- m. NUX-M. PETR. Phos. Psor. Stram. Sulph. Valer. Verat.

MOANING — Acon. Apis. Ars. Bar-c. BELL. Bry. Calad. Camph.CANN-I. Carb- ac. Cham. Cic. Cina. Cocc. Colch. Crot-c. Cupr. Eup-per. Gels. Hyos. Ign. Ip. Kali-br. KALI-C. Lach. Merc. Mur-ac.

Nit-ac. Nux-v. OP. Phos. Podo. PULS. Sec. Stram. Sulph. Verat. ZINC.

MOROSE—Agar. Am-c. ANAC. Aran. Arn. Art-v. AUR. Bell. Bism. Bry. Calc. Caust. Colch. Coloc. Con. Crot-t. Cycl. Dig. Ferr. Ferr-p. Guai. Ip. KALI-P. Led. Lyc. Merc. Mez. Mur-ac. NUX-V. Phos-ac. Phos. Plat. Plb. PULS. SIL. Stry. Sulph. Thuj. Valer. Verb. Zinc.

OBSTINATE— Acon. Agar. Aloe. ALUM. ANAC. Arg- n. Ars. BELL. Bry. Calc. Caps. Cham. Chin. Cina. Dig. Ferr. Hep. Ign. kali-p. Kreos. Lach. Lyc. Mag-m. Merc. Nit-ac. NUX-V. Pall. Phos-ac. Psor. Sil. Spong. Stram. SULPH. TARENT. Thuj. Viol-o. Zinc.

QUARRELSOME— Anac. Ars. AUR. Bell. Brom. Bry. Camph. Canth. Caust. CHAM. Con. Croc. Cupr. Dulc. Hyos. IGN. Kali-c. Lach. Lyc. Merc. Mosch. Nat-c. Nat-m. Nit- ac. NUX-V. PETR. Phos-ac.

Phos. Plat. Psor. Sep. **Staph.**
STRAM. SULPH. TARENT.
Thuj. Verat. Verat-v. Viol-t. **Zinc.**

RECOGNISE, DOES
NOT, HIS RELATIVES—
Acet-ac. Agar. **Anac. BELL.**
Calad. Cic. Cupr. **Glon. Hyos.**
Kali-bi, **Lach. Meli. Merc.**
Oena. **OP.** Phos. Plb, Sulph-ac.
Tab. Valer. **Verat.** Zinc.

    ,,   OWN HOUSE—
Meli. Merc. Psor.

    ,,   WELL-KNOWN
STREETS—Cann-I. **Glon.**
Lach. **NUX-M. PETR.**

RESTLESSNESS—
ACON. Agar. **ARG-N.** Arn.
ARS. Ars-i. Art-v. Asaf. **Aur.**
Aur-m. **Bapt. BELL.** Bov. Calc.
Calc-p. Camph. Caust. Carb-v.
Cimic. Cit-v. Coloc. Cupr.
Cup-ars. FERR. Ferr-ars.
HYOS. Kali-br. Kali-c. **Lach.**
Lyc. **Merc.** Mosch. Nat-m. Op.
Phos. Plb. Psor. **PULS. RHUS-**
T. Sec. Sep. **Sil. Staph.**
STRAM. SULPH. TARENT.
Thuj. **VALER.** Verat. Vip.
ZINC.

RUDENESS— Arn. **Aur.**
Bell. Canth.Graph. **Hyos.** Lac-
c. **LYC. Nit-ac. Nux-v.** Op.
Phos. **Stram. VERAT.**

STARTING—Arn. Ars-i.
Bar-c. **BELL. Bor. Bry.** Bufo
Calc. **CAPS.** Carb-an. Carb-s.
Carb-v. Caust. **Cic.** Cocc. **Con.**
Cur. Graph. Hura **HYOS.** Ign.
Kali-ars. **KALI-C.** Kali-i. **Kali-p.**
Kali-s. **LAC-C.** Lach. Lyc. **Med.**
Mur-ac. **Nat-ar.** Nat-c. **NAT-M.**
Nat-p. **Nit-ac. Nux-m. Nux-v.**
Op. Petr. **Phos.** Sep. Sil. **STRAM.**
STRON-MET. Stry. Sulph.
Ther. Verat. Zinc.

STUPEFACTION—
APIS. Ars.**BAPT. Bell.** Bry. Cic.
Cocc. Cupr. Ferr. **GELS.**
HELL. HYOS. Kali-p. Lyc.
Mag-m. **NUX-V. OP.** Petr.
PHOS-AC. Phos. Plb. Puls.
Rhus-t. Sep. **STRAM.** Sulph.
Thuj. **Verat.** Vinc. **Zinc.**

VIOLENT—Acon.
Anac. Ars. **AUR.** Bar-c. **BELL.**
Bry. Carb-V. **Cham. CIC.** Cupr.
Graph. Hep. **HYOS. Kali-p.**
Lach. Lyc. Mosch. **Nat-m.** Nit-

ac. **NUX-V.** Petr. **Phos.** Plat. Sep. **STRAM.** Sulph. Tarent. Verat. **Visc.**

WEARY OF LIFE—Ant-c. **ARS. AUR.** Bell. Caust. **Chin.** Hep. Hyos. **Kali-p.** Lach. Lyc. Merc. **Nat-m. NIT-AC. Nux-v. PHOS.** Plb. **Puls.** Rhus-t. Sep. Sil. Staph. Stram. Sulph. Thuj. Valer. Verat.

WORK, AVERSION TO MENTAL—**ALOE.** Anac. **Aur. BAPT. BROM. Calc.** Carb-ac. **Chel. CHIN.** Chinin-ar. Colch. Ferr. **Gels.** Hyos. Kali-bi. **KALI-P.** Lach. **LEC. Lyc.** Med. Mur-ac. **Nat-m.** Nit-ac. **NUX-V.** Op. **Phos-ac. PHOS.** Phyt. **PIC-AC.** Plat. **Puls.** Rhus-t. **Sep. Sil.** Staph. **Sulph.** Thuj. Tub. Valer.

WRONG, EVERY-THING SEEMS—Coloc. Eug.Hep. **Naja** Nux-v.

VERTIGO

Acon.**AGAR.** Ail. Apis. **ARG-M.** Arg-n. Ars. **Aur.** Bapt. **BRY. Calc.** Calc-s. **Cann-I.** Carb-s. **Chel. CHIN. Chin-s.** Cic. **COCC. CON. Cycl. Dig.** Dulc. Ferr. **GELS.** Ip. Kali-c. **KALI-P.** Lach. **LYC.** Merc. Mosch. **Nat-c. NAT-M.** Nat-s. Op. **Petr. Phos-ac. PHOS.** Plat. Psor. **Pic-ac. PULS. Rhus-t. Sang.** Sec. **SIL.** Spig. Stann. Stram. **SULPH. TAB.** Ther. Thuj. **Valer.** Verat. **Verat-v.** Zinc.

MORNING — Am-c. **Arg-n.** Bov. **Bry.** Calc. **CARB-AN.** Carb-s. Chel. **Chin.** Dulc. Gels. Kali-c. Kali-p. **LACH. LYC.** Mag-c. **Nat-m.** Nat-p. **NUX-V.** Petr. **Phos.ac. Phos.** Puls.Sep. Sil. Sulph. Verat. Zinc.

FORE-NOON —Agar. Bry. Calc. Carb-v. **Caust.** Cham.Chin-s. Eup.per. Fl-ac.Lach.Lacc. **Lyc. Nat-m. Phos.** Samb. Sars. Stann. **Sulph.** Viol-t. Zinc.

NOON—Aeth. Arn. **Calc-p. Caust.** Chin. Dulc. Harm. Kalm. lyc. Mag-s. Merc. Nat-s. Nux-v. Phos. Stram. Sulph. Zinc.

AFTER-NOON—**AEsc.** Agar. Alum. **Ambr.** Benz-ac. **Bry.**

Carb-s. Chel. **Chin.** Cupr. Cycl. Dios. Ferr. Ferr-p. **Glon.** Hura. Kali-c. **Kali-p. LYC.** Merc. Nat-m. Nux-v. Phos-ac. **Phos.** Puls. Rhus-t. **Sep.** Sil. Staph. Sulph. Thuj.

EVENING—Alum. **Am-c.** Apis. **ARS.** Bor. **CALC. Carb-s.** Carb-v. Chin. **Cycl.** Dios. Graph. Hep.Iris. Kali-ar. **Kali-p.** Kali-s. **Lach.** Lyc. Mag-c. Merc. Nat-m. Nat-s. **Nit-ac.** Nux-m. **Nux-v.** Phos-ac. **PHOS.** Pic-ac. **PULS.** Rhod. Selen. Sep. **Sil.** Staph. **Sulph.** Thuj. Zinc.

NIGHT—**Am-c.** Bell. Calc. Caust. **Chin.** Croc. **Cycl.** Dig. Ham. Lac-c. **Lach.** Nat-c. **Nux-v. PHOS.** Pic-ac. Rhod. Sang. **Sil. Spong.** Stram. Sulph.Ther. **Thuj.** Zinc.

ASCENDING STAIRS— Ant-c. Bor. **CALC.** Carb-ac. Coca. Glon. **Kali-bi.** Merc. Pic-ac. Sulph.

CLOSING EYES ON— **Alum.** Alumn. Ant-t. Apis. **Arg-n. ARN.** Ars. **CHEL.** Cycl. Ferr.

Hep. **LACH.** Mag-s. petr. Phos-ac. **Pip-m. SEP.** Sil. **Stram. THER.** Thuj. Zinc.

"   AMEL—Alum. **Con.** Dig. Ferr. **Gels.** Graph. **Pip-m.** Sel. Sulph. **TAB.** VERAT-V.

COFFEE AFTER — Arg-n. **Cham.** Mosch. **NAT-M.** Nux-v. Phos.

COITION AFTER — **Phos-ac.** Sep.

CROSSING   A BRIDGE—Bar-c. Brom.

" RUNNING WATER — **Ang. Arg-m.** Brom. Ferr. Sulph.

DESCENDING, ON— BOR. Coff. Con.**FERR.** Gels. Mag-m. Sanic. Stann.

"   STAIRS—BOR. Carb-ac. **Con.** Gins. Merl. Merc. Phys. **Plat.** Tarent.

DINNER, AFTER— Aloe. Bell. Coloc. Ferr. **Hep. Mag-s.** Nat-s. **NUX-V.** Petr. Phos. Puls. Sel. **Sulph.** Thuj. **Zinc.**

EATING, WHILE — Am-c. Calc. Con. Dios. **GRAT.**

Mag-c. Nat-c. **Nux-v. Phos.** Sel. Sil.

"   **AFTER** — Alum. Bry. **Cham.** Chin. cocc. Cycl. **GRAT. Kali-bi.** Kali-c. Kali-p. **Lach.** Lyc. Mag-s. **Nat-s. Nux-v.** Petr. **Phos. Puls.** Rhus-t. Sep. **Sulph.** Tarent. Zinc.

HEADACHE, DURING —**Acon.** Anac. **APIS Arg-n.** Arn. **Ars. Aur.** Bar-c. **BELL.** Bov. Bry. **CALC. Calc-p.** Caust. Chel. Coff. **Con.** Cupr. Ferr. **Ferr-p. Gels. GLON.** Hep. Kali-bi. Kali-br. **Kali-c.** Kalm. **Lach.** Mag-m. Merc. **Nat-m. Nat-s.** Nux-m. **Nux-v.** Phos. Plb. Psor. **Puls. SANG.** Sep. **SIL.** Spig. Strontmet. Sulph. Tab. **Verat-v.** Zinc.

LOOKING DOWNWARD—Alumn. Calc. Con. Ferr. **Kalm.** Mag-m. Nat-c. Nux-v. Petr. **PHOS.** Puls. Sep. **SPIG.** Staph. **SULPH.** Thuj.

"   **STEADILY**—Am-c. **Caust.** Cur. **Kali-c.** Lach. **NAT-M.** Phos. Sil. Spig. Sulph. Tarent.

"   **UPWARDS—Calc.** Carb-v. **Caust.** Cupr. Dig. Graph. Iod. Kali-p. Lach. Mur-ac. **Nux-v.** Petr. **PHOS. Plb. Puls.** Sang. Sep. Sil. **Tab.** Thuj.

"   **WINDOW, OUT OF A**—Camph. **Carb-v. NAT-M.** Ox-ac.

MENTAL EXERTION —**Agar.** Am-c. **Arg-n.** Bar-c. Bor. Calc. Coff. Kalm. **NAT-C. NAT-M.** Nat-p. **NUX-V. Phos-ac.** Pic-ac. **Puls.** Sep. Sil. **Staph.**

NAUSEA, WITH— **ACON.** Alum. **Alumn.** Am-c. **Ant-c.** Bapt. Bar-c. **Bell. BRY.** Calc. **Calc-p.** Calc-s. **Camph.** Carb-an. Carb-v. Caust. Cham. Chel. **CHININ-S.** Cinnb. **COCC.** Con. **Cycl. FERR.** Ferr-ar. **Glon.** Graph. Ham. Hell. Hep. Ind. **Kali-bi.** Kali-p. Kalm. Lac-c. **Lach. LOB.** Lyc. Lyss. Merc. Mosch. **Nat-m.** Nit-ac. **NUX-V. PETR. Phos. Puls.** Rhus-t. Sang. **Sep.** Sil. Spig. Staph. Sulph. **Tab.** Ther. Verat. **Verat-v.** zinc.

OBJECTS SEEM TO TURN IN A CIRCLE—Agar. Alum. Bar-c **Bry. CHEL.** Cic. Cocc. Colch. Con. Cycl. Kali-c. Kali-p. Lyc. Mag-c. Mur-ac. **NAT-M.** Nat-s. **Nux-v.** Op. Phos-ac. **Psor.** Rhus-t. Sep. Sil. Sulph-ac.

PERIODICAL—Agar. **Arg-m.** Camph. **Cocc.** Cycl.**Ign.** Kali-c. **NAT-M. PHOS.** Tab. Ust.

RAISING HEAD— Acon. Ant-t. **Arn.** Bar-c. **BRY.** Calc.**Carb-v. CHIN.** Croc. Laur. Mag-s. **Nux-v.** Op. **Phos. Pic.ac.** Sel. Stann. Stram.

RIDING, WHILE— Ant-t.Dig. Grat.

" IN A CARRIAGE— Acon. Calc. **Hep.** Lyc. Sel. Sil.

" AMEL — Glon. Sil. RISING. ON — ACON. Ail. Aml-ns. Arn. Bar-c. **Bell. BRY.** Calc. **Cann-I. Carb-an.** Caust. Chin. Cic. Con. Dig. **FERR.**Ferr-p. **Glon.** Guai. Ham. Hyos. Kali-bi. Kali-p. Lac-d. **Lach.** Merc. **NAT-M.** Nux-v. Petr. **PHOS.**

Puls. **RHUS-T.** Sil. Sulph. **TAB.** Thuj. Verat-v.

" FROM BED ON— **Agar.** Arn. Bar-c. **Bell. BRY. Cact. CHEL.** Chin. Cimi. **COCC.** Dulc. **FERR. Ferr-p.** Fl-ac. **Glon.** Kali-bi. Lyc. Mag-m. **NUX-V.** Op. Petr. **Phos-ac. PHOS. PHYT.** Pic-ac. Puls. Rhus.t. **Sep.** Sil. Stram. Sulph. Verat-v.

SLEEP, DURING— Aeth. Crot-h. **Lyc. Sang. Sep. Sil,** Ther.

SLEEP, AFTER, AGG— Ambr. Ars. **Calc.** Carb-v. **Chin.** Dulc. **Graph.** Hep. **Kali-p.** Kali-i. **LACH.** Lact. **Med.** Nat-m. **NUX-V.** Op. **Sep.** Spong. Stram. **Ther.** Thuj. Zinc.

STAGGERING, WITH — Alis-p. **Arg-n. Aur.** Bry. Calc. Camph. Carb-an. **Carb-v.** Cham. Chin. **Cic. CON.** Ferr.**GELS.** Ign.Kali-br. Lyc. Mur-ac. **Nux-m. NUX-V.** Petr. **PHOS.** Phyt. Sep. **Stram.** Sulph. Thuj.

STOOPING, ON —
Alum. Anac. Arg-n. Aur. Bar-c. **BELL. BRY.** Calc-p. Camph. Carb-v. **Caust.** Cham. Con. Dig. **Glon.** Graph. Guare. Ham. Hell. **Ign.** Iod. **Kali-bi.** Kali-p. Kalm. **Lach.** Lyc. Merc-c. Mosch. Nat-m. Nit-ac. **NUX-V.** Petr, **Phos. PULS.** Sep. Sil. **Staph, SULPH.** Ther. Valer.

SYNCOPE, WITH —
Alum. Ars. **Bry.** Canth. Carb-v. Cham. Croc. **GLON.** Hep. **Lach.** Mag.c. Mosch. **NUX-V.** Phos. Sulph.

SYPHILITIC — AUR.

TEA, ATFER — NAT-M. SEP.

"   AMEL — Glon.

TURNING IN BED, ON — **BELL. Cact.** Carb-v. **CON. Graph.** Ind. Kalm. **Lac-d.** Meph. Phos. Rhus-t. Sulph.

VISION, OBSCU-RATION OF WITH—Acon. **Anac.** Arg-n. **Bell.** Calc. Camph. **CYCL.** Dulc. **FERR. FERR-**AR. GELS. GLON,** Hep. **Kali-bi.** Lach.Merc. **Nit-ac. NUX-V.** Par. **PHOS.** Phyt. Puls. **Sabin. Stram.** Stron-met. Sulph. Tereb. Zinc.

VOMITING, WITH —
Ars. Calc. Canth. Chel. Crot-t. **Glon. Graph.** Hell. **KALI-BI,** Kali-c. **Lach.** Mag-c Merc. Mosch. **Nat-s. Nux-v.**

WALKING, WHILE —
Apis. **Arg-n.** Bell. **Bry.** Calc. Cann-I. Cocc. **Con.** Dulc. **Ferr.** Ferr-i. **Gels.** Hell. Hyos. Ign. Kali-bi. Kali-c. Kali-p. Laur. Mag-m. **Mur-ac. NAT-M.** Nat-s. Nit-ac. **Nux-m. Nux-v.** Petr. Phel. Phos-ac. **PHOS.** Phyt. Pic-ac. **Psor. PULS. Rhus-t.** Sec. **Sep. Sil.** Spig. **Stram. Sulph.** Tarent. Thuj, Verat. Zinc.

NIGHT WATCHING AND LOSS OF SLEEP, FROM – COCC. NUX-V.

WINDY WEATHER— Calc-p.

HEAD

BALANCING SENSATION IN — Aesc. Bell. **Glon.** Lyc.

BOARD OR BAR BEFORE, SENSATION AS OF A — Acon. Aesc. Calc. **Carb-an.** Cocc. **Dulc.** Helon. Kreos. Lyc. Op. Plat. Plb. **RHUS-T.** Sulph. Znc.

BOILING SENSATION IN —ACON. Cann-I. Coff. DIG. Graph. Hell. Kali-c. Lyc. Mag-m. Merc. Sil. Sulph.

BORES HEAD IN PILLOW — APIS. Arn. BELL. **Bry.** Camph. Crot-t. Dig. HELL. Hyper. MED. STRAM. Sulph. Tarent. TUB.

CEREBRAL HEMORRHAGE—ACON. ARN. **Aur.** Bar-c. BELL. Camph. **CARB-V. Chin. Coff.** Colch. Con. **Cupr. Crot-h. Ferr. GELS.** Hyos. **Ip. Lach.** Laur. Lyc. Merc. Nat-m. Nit-ac. **Nux-m. Nux-v. OP. Phos.** Plb. **Puls.** Stram.

CONGESTION—

ACON. Am-br. Anac. Ant-c. Apis. **Arg-n. ARN.** Ars. **Aur.** BELL. Bor. Bry. Bufo. **CACT. Calc.** Calc-p. Calc-s. Camph. Cann-s. **Canth.** Carb-an. **Carb-s. CARB-V.** Cham. Chin. **Cimic.** Cocc. Croc. **CUPR.** Cycl. **Dulc. FERR. FERR-P.** Fl-ac. **GELS. GLON.** Graph. **Hell. Hyos.** Iod. Kali-bi. **Kali-br.** Kali-c. Kali-i. Kali-p. **LACH.** Laur. **Lyc.** Mag-s. **MELI.** Merc. Mill. **Nat-c. NAT-M. Nux-v. OP.** Phos-ac. **PHOS.** Pic-ac. Plb. Psor. Puls. Ran-b. **Rhus-t. SANG.** Sep. Sil. Spong. **Stram. Stry. SULPH.** Sulph-ac. Tab. Thuj. Urt-u. **Verat. Verat-v.** Zinc.

ENLARGED SENSATION—AGAR. Apis **ARG-N. ARN.** Ars. Bapt. **BELL.** Berb. Bov. Cact. Caps. **Cimic.** Cor-r. Dulc. Echi. Gels. **GLON.** Hyper. Kali-i. Lac-d. Lach. Mang. Merc. **Nat-m. NUX-M. NUX-V.** Par. Plat. **RAN-B.** Sil. **Spig.** Sulph. Ther. Verat.

FULNESS, AS IF IT WOULD BURST — Am-c. aster. **Cann-I.** Daph. **GLON.** Ip. Lil-t. Merc. Nit-ac.

HANDS. HOLDS HEAD, WITH—**GLON.** Hyos.

" ON COUGHING— BRY. Nicc. **NUX-V.** Sulph.

HAT, AVERSION TO—Carb-an. **Iod.** Led. **Lyc.**

HEADACHE

HEADACHE—**ACON.** Am-c. **Anthr-aci. Apis** Arg-m. **ARG-N.** Arn. **ARS. AUR.** Bapt. **BELL.** Bor. **BRY. Calc.** Calc-p. Calc-s. Carb-v. Cham. **Cocc. Crot-c.** Cupr. Dig. **FERR-P.** Gels. **GLON.** Graph. **HEL. Hyos.** Ign. **IRIS. Kali-bi.** Kali-c. **KALI-I.** Kali-p. Kali-s. Kalm. **LACH,** Lyc. **Mag-p. MERC.** Nat-c. **NAT-M. Nat-s. NIT-AC.** Nux-m. **NUX-V.** Op. Rhus-t. **SANG. Sep. SIL. Spig. SULPH.** Tereb. Thuj. Verat. **VERAT-V.** Zinc,

AIR, OPEN, AMEL.— Alum. **Apis. ARS.** Aur. **Bell.** Cann-I. **Carb-v.** Cimic. **Ferr. GLON.** Hell. Hyos. **Kali-bi.** Kali-i. Kali-P. **KALI-S.** Led. **Lyc.** Mag-m. **MANG.** Mez. **Nat-m.** Op. **PHOS. PULS. Sang.** Sel. **Seneg. SEP.** Sulph. Tab. **ZINC.**

ASCENDING STEPS, ON—Arn. **BELL. BRY. CALC. Carb-v.** Cupr. Ferr. **Gels. Glon.** Ign. Kalm. **Lach.** Lyc. Meph. **Mosch.** Nux-v. Phos-ac. **Phos.** Psor. **Rhns-t.** Sang. **Sep. SIL. SPONG.** Sulph. Tab. Zinc.

BINDING HEAD, AMEL—Apis. **Arg-m. ARG-N.** Arn. **Bell. BRY. Calc.** Carb-ac. **Hep.** Lac-d. **Mag-m.** Nux-v. Pic-ac. Psor. **PULS.** Rhod. **SIL.** Spig.

BLINDING— Asar. Aster. **Bell. Caust. CYCL.** Ferr-p. **GELS, IRIS. Lac-d.** Lil-t. **Nat-m.** Petr. Phos. **Psor. SIL.** Stram. Sulph.

BLOWING NOSE, AGG.— Ambr. Aster. **AUR.**

BELL. Calc. **Chel.** Ferr. **HEP.** Mur-ac. Nit-ac. **PULS. SULPH.**

CLOSING EYE, ON, AMEL—Acon. Agar. Aloe **BELL. BRY.** Calc. Chel. Coff. Con. Hell. Hyos. Ign. Iod. Ip. Nat-m. Nux-v. Plat. Rhus t. **Sep. SIL. Spig. Sulph. Zinc.**

COLD APPLICATIONS, AMEL — Acon. ALOE. Am-c. Ant-c. **ARS. Bell.** Bry. Calc. Calc-p. Cham. **Euph.** Ferr. **Ferr-p. GLON.** Iod. Kali-bi. Lac-d. **LACH.** Led. Mosch. **NAT-M. PHOS.** Psor. **PULS.** Spig. **Stram. SULPH.** Zinc.

CONSTIPATED WHILE—Aloe Alum. **BRY. Calc-p.** Coff. **Coll.** Con. Crot-h. Ign. **Lac-d.** Lach. Mag-c. **Nat-m. Nat-s. NUX-V.** OP. **Plb.** Petr. **Podo. Puls.** Verat. Zinc.

EATING, AFTER—Agar. Alum. Ars. **Bry.** Calc. **Calc-p.** Calc.s. **Carb-v.** Cham. **Cocc.** Coff. Con. Dios. Ferr. Ferr-p. Gels. Glon. **Graph.** Hyos. Kali-c. Lach. **Lyc.** Mag-c. **NAT-C.**

NAT-M. Nux-m. **NUX-V.** Petr. **Phos-ac.** Phos. **PULS.** Rhus-t. Sep. Sil. **SULPH.** Verat. Zinc.

EPISTAXIS, AMEL.— Ant-c. Bufo. Carb-an. Cham. Dig. Ferr-p. Ham. Hyos. Kali-bi. Mag-s. **MEL.** Mill. **Petr. Psor.** Tab.

FOOT-STEPS. AGG.—COFF. NUX-V. Sil.

HAMMERING — Am-C. Ars. Aur. **BELL.** Chin. **Chinin-s.** Cimic. **Cocc.** Coff. **Cur. FERR. FERR-AR.** Ferr-p. **GLON.** Hep. Iris. Kali-i. **Lach.** Mag-s. Mez. **NAT-M.** Nit-ac. Psor. Puls. Rhus-t. **SIL. SULPH.** Tarent.

HAT FROM PRESSURE OF—Agar. Alum. Arg-m. **Calc-p.** Carb-an. **CARB-V.** Caust. Crot-t. Ferr-i. **GLON.** Hep. Kali-n. Lach. Laur. Led. Lyc. Mez. **NIT-AC.** Sep. Sil. Staph. Sulph. **Valer.**

HOT DRINKS, AGG—Arum-t. PHOS. PULS. Sulph.

INCREASING AND

DECREASING GRADUALLY
—Arn. Ars. Bar-c. Crot-h. Glon.
Mez. Nat-m. Op. Pic-ac. **Plat.**
Psor. Sars. Spig. **STANN.** Staph.
Sulph. Verb.

IRONING, FROM—
BRY.

JAR, FROM ANY—Arn.
BELL. BRY. Calc. **Carb-v.**
Carb.s. Chin. Crot-h. **Ferr-p.**
Gels. **GLON.** Hep.Kali-c.Kali-
s. Lac-d. **Lach. LED.** Lyc. Mag-
m. Merc. **Nat-m. NIT-AC.**
Nux-v. Petr. **Phos-ac. Phos.** Psor.
Rhus-t. San. Sep. SIL. Spig.
Sulph. Ther. **Thuj.** Vib.

LIES WITH HEAD
HIGH—Arg-m. **ARS.** Bry. Carb-
v. **Con. Gels.** Nat-m. **Phos.**
PULS. Spig. Stron-met.

MOTION FROM—
Anac. **Ant-c.** Apis. **BELL. BRY.**
Calc-p. Caps. **CARB-V. Carb-s.**
Chin. **Cimic.** Cocc. **Coff. con.**
Crot-t. Ferr-p. Gels. GLON.
HEP. Ign. Kali-bi. **Kreos.** Lac-d.
Lach. LED. Lyc. Mag-m. **Mag-**
p. Mang. **Meli. MEZ. Mosch.**
Nat-m. NIT-AC. Nux-m.

Nux-v. Phos-ac.**Phos.** Pso
Rumex. **Sang.** Sars. Sep. Sil. **Spig**
Stann. Staph. Sulph. **Ther.** Vera

AMEL.—**Agar.** Arg-m
Ars. Benz-ac. **Caps.** Cham. Co
Ferr. Hyos. Ign. **Iris.** Kali-p. **Ly**
Magm. **Mur-ac.** Nat-c. **Nux-m**
Puls. Rhod. **RHUS-T.** Stann
Valer.

PERIODIC HEAD
ACHE— Aeth. Aloe **ALUM**
Anac. Apis. **ARS.** Ars-i. Bell. **Cac**
Calc. Carbv. **CEDR. CHIN**
Chinin-ar.   CHININ-S
COLOC. Cupr. Eup-per. **Fer**
Ferr-ar. **Ign.** Kali-ar. **KALI-B**
Kreos. Lac-d. **Lach.** Lyc. **NAT**
M. **NIT-AC.** Nux-v. **Phos**
Puls. Rhus-t. **SANG.** Sel. **SE**
SIL. Spig. **Stram.** Sulph. **Tu**
Zinc.

PRESSURE, AMEL.–
Alumn. **AM-C.** Anac. Apis. Ar
m. **Arg-n. BELL. BRY.** Cal
Chin. Cinnb. **Coloc. FER**
Ferr-i. **Ferr-p. Glon.** Hell. I
Kali-bi. Lac-d. **LACH.** Ly
Mag-c. **MAG-M. MAG-P.** Me
NAT-M. Nat-s. Nux-v. Pho

Pic-ac. **Puls.** Pyrog. **Rhus-t. Sang.** Sep. **Sil. Spig. STANN.** Sulph. Thuj. Verat. Zinc.

READING AGG.—Arg-m. Aur. Bry. **Calc.** Carb-v. Cham. Cimic. Coff. Ferr-i. **Glon. Lach.** Lyc. **NAT-M.** Nat-s. **NUX-V.** Op. **Phos-ac. Plat.** Ruta Sep. Sil. Sulph. **Tub.**

SLEEP, AMEL.—Bell. Chel. Colch. Ferr. **Gels. Glon.** Graph.Hyos. Lac-c. **Pall. PHOS.** Pic-ac. Puls. **Sang. Sep.**

STOOPING, FROM— Alum. Apis. Bar-c. **BELL. BRY.** Calc. Chel. Cocc. **Coff. Coloc.** Dig. Dulc. Ferr. **Ferr-p.** Ign. Kali-c. Kali-n. kali-s. Lach. Led. **MANG. MERC. Nat-m.** Nat-s. **Nit-ac. Nux-m. NUX-V.** Petr. Phos. **PULS.** Rhus-t. **Sang.** Seneg. **SEP.** Sil. **SPIG.** Stann. **SULPH.** Thuj. **VALER.** Verat.

SUN FROM EXPOSURE TO—ACON. Agar. Aloe. **ANT-C.** Arum-t. Bar-c. **BELL. BRY.** Calc. Camph. Carb-v. Chin. Cocc. **Gels. Glon.** Hyos. Ign. **LACH. NAT-C.** Nat-

m. Nux-v. **PULS. Sel. Stram.** Sulph. **Ther.** Valer. Zinc.

TALKING WHILE— Acon. Aran. Arg-n. **Aur. BELL.** Bry. Calc. Calc-s. Chin. Cocc. Fl-ac. **Gels. Glon. Ign.** Iod. Jug-r. **Lac-c. Mag-m.** Meli. Mez. **NAT-M.** Nux-v. Phos-ac. Puls. Rhus-t. Sang. **Sil.** Spig. **SULPH.** Zinc.

UNCONSCIOUSNESS, WITH—Acon. Arg-n. **BELL.** Bov. Cann-I. **Crot-h.** Ferr. **GLON.** Iod. Kali-c. Mag-c. **Mosch. NAT-M. Verat.**

WALKING, WHILE, AMEL.—Am-c. Calc. **Cycl.** Gels. **Guai.** Hyos. **LYC.** Mur-ac. Nat-c. Nat-m. **PHOS.** Puls. **RHOD. RHUS-T.** Sep. Staph. Sulph. **Tarax. Thuj.**

WARM BED, IN— BELL. **Carb-v. LYC. MEZ.**

WINE, FROM—Ant-c. **Ars.** Bell. Calc. **Carb-an. Carb-v.** Con. **Gels. Glon.** Ign. Lach. **Led.** Lyc. **Nat-c.** Nat-m. **NUX-V. Oxac.** Petr. Ran-b. Rhod. **SEL. Sil.** Stron-met. Verat. **ZINC.**

WRAPPING UP HEAD, AMEL.—Arg-n. **Ars. Aur. Bell.** Bry. colch. Con. Cupr. **Gels.** HEP. Kali-c. Kali-i. Lach. **Mag-m. Mag-p.** Mez. **Nit-ac. Nux-m. NUX-V.** Phos-ac. **RHOD. RHUS-T.** Sanic. **Sep. SIL.** Squil. Stron-met. Thuj.

EYE

BLEEDING IN THE RETINA (RETINAL HEMORRHAGE)—Arn. BELL. Crot-h. Glon. Ham. LACH. Merc-c. Phos. Prun. Sulph.

BLURRED VISION— Ars. **Aur.** Cact. Calc. **Con.** Crot-c. GELS. Glon. Kali-p. LAC-C. Lil-t. **Lyc.** Med. **NAT-M.** Nux-v. Phos. **Phys.** Plat. **Psor.** Rhus-t. **Ruta** Stram. Teucr. Thuj.

BURNING PAIN, IN— ACON. Agar. All-c. ALUM. Am-m. APIS. Arg-n. ARS. Aur. Bell. Bry. **Calc. Canth. Caps.** Carb-s. CARB-V. Caust. Chel. CHIN. Clem. CON. Crot-h. Crot-t. Dios. EUPHR. Ferr-p.

Glon. **Graph.** Hep. Iod. **Kali-bi. Kali-c.** Kali-s. LACH. Lyc. Mag-m. **Merc. MERC-C.** Nat-c. **NAT-M. Nat-s. Nit-ac.** Nux-v. Op. Petr. PHOS-AC. **Phos. Puls.** RAN-B. Rhus-t. **RUTA Sang.** Sep. SULPH. Tarent. Thuj. Verat. Zinc.

DIPLOPIA— Agar. **Aluma.** Arg-n. **AUR. BELL.** Cann-I. **Caust. Chel.** Cic. **con. Cycl.** Daph. **Dig. GELS.** Graph. HYOS. Iod. **Kali-c. kali-cy. Lyc. Lyss.** Merc. **Merc-c. Morph.** NAT-M. Nicc. NIT-AC. Nux-v. Op. **Plb.** Puls. Seneg. Stann. **STRAM.** Sulph. Ther. Thuj. Verat. Zinc.

INJECTED—Acon. All-c. Ant-t. Arg-n. BELL. Camph. **Clem.** Con. Ferr. FERR-P. Gels. GLON. Hep. **Kali-bi.** Kali-s. Lach. **Merc.** NAT-M. NUX-V. OP. Phos. STRAM. Sulph. Zinc.

SEES HALOS OF COLORS AROUND THE LIGHT—Alum. Anac. Bar-c. BELL. Bry. Calad. Calc. **Carb-v.**

Chin. Cic. **Cycl. Dig.** Gels. Hep. Ip. Kali-c. **Lach.** Mag-m. **Nicc.** Nit-ac. **OSM. Phos-ac. PHOS. PULS.** Ruta Sars. Sep. Staph. **SULPH.** Tub. Zinc.

EARS

NOISES IN—Ambr. Arg-n. **Ars. Aur.** Bar-c. **BELL. Bor.** Cact. **CALC. CANN-I.** Caust. **CHIN. CHININ-S.** Cupr. Ferr-p. **GRAPH.** Kali-c. **KALI-I.** Kali-p. Kali-s. Kreos. **Lach. LYC.** Lyss. **Merc.** Nat-m. **Nat-s.** Nux-v. Op. **PETR. Phos-ac.** Plat. Plb. **Psor. PULS.** Rhod. **SANG.** Sil. **SPIG.** Staph. Stram. **SULPH.** Tab. Thuj. **TUB.** Valer. Verat. Xanth. Zinc.

NOSE

BLOOD, CONGESTION OF, IN THE — Am-c. Calc. **CUPR.** Samb. **Sulph.**

EPISTAXIS —**ACON.** Agar. Alumn. **Ambr. AM-C. Ant-c. ARN.** Ars. Bapt. **BELL. Both. Bov.** Bry. **CACT.** Calc.

Calc-p. Calc-s. **Carb-s. CARB-V. Caust.** Chin. **CROC. CROT-H. Cupr.** Dros. Elaps. **Glon. HAM. Hyos.** Ip. **Kali-i. Kali-p. LACH.** Lyc. **Med. MELI. MERC. MILL.** Nat-c. Nat-m. **NIT-AC. NUX-V.** Phos-ac. **PHOS. PULS. Rhus-t. Sabin.** Sang. **SEC.** Stann. **SULPH.** Sulph-ac. Thuj. **TUB.** Ust. **Verat.** Zinc.

REDNESS OF THE— Aloe. **ALUM. Ars.** Apis. **Aur. Bar-c. Bell.** Bor. Calc. Carb-v. Caust. **CHIN.** Fl-ac. Graph. Hep. **Kali-bi. Kali-c. Lach.** Led. **Mag-m.** Merc. **Merc-c. Nat-c.** Nat-m. **PHOS.** Plb. Rhus-t **SULPH.** Thuj. **Zinc.**

FACE

BLOATED—**ACON.** Ant-t. **APIS. APOC. ARS. Aur. Bell.** Bry. Camph. **Chin.** Cocc. Colch. **Crot-h.** Dig. **Dulc.** glon. Hippoz. Hyos. **Kali-c. Lach. Merc. Nat-m. Op. Phos. Puls.** Samb. Sep. Sulph. **Vesp.**

BLUISH—Apis. Arg-n. ARS. Asaf. BAPT. BELL. Bry. CAMPH. Cann-I. CARB-V. Chlor. Con. CUPR. DIG. Glon. HYOS. Ip. Kali-cy. LACH. Laur. Lyc. MORPH. Nat-m. Op. Phos. Puls. Staph. SULPH. VERAT. VERAT-V. Vip. Zinc.

DROPPING OF THE JAW—Acet-ac. Apis. Arn. Ars. Bapt. Carb-v. Chel. Cupr. Gels. Glon. Hell. HYOS. Kali-i. LACH. LYC. Merc-cy. MUR-AC. Nux-v. Op. Phos-ac. Phos. Podo. Sec. Stram. SULPH. Verat-v. Zinc.

PALE—Anac. ANT-T. Apis ARG-M. ARS. Aur. Bell. Berb. CALC. CALC-P. Calc-s. CAMPH. Canth. Carb-an. Carb-s. CARB-V. Caust. CHIN. Chinin-s. CINA Clem. DIG. FERR. Ferr-i. FERR-P. GRAPH. Hyos. Kali-c. Lob. Lyc. Mang. Med. Nat-ar. Nat-c. NAT-M. Nat-p. Op. PHOS-AC. PLB. Puls. SEC. SEP. Sulph. TAB. Tub. VERAT. Vip. ZINC.

RED—ACON. Apis. AML-NS. Arg-n. Aur. BAPT. BELL. bry. Caps. Chel. Chin. Cic. Cina Crot-h. dig. FERR. FERR-I. GLON. HYOS. Kali-i. LACH. MELI. Merc. Mez. Naja NUX-V. OP. Phos. Rhus-t. SANG. Sil. STRAM. Sulph. Terb. Verat-v.

WRINKLED FOREHEAD—Acet-ac. Alum. Brom. Caust. Cham. Cycl. Graph. Hell. LYC. Merc. Nat-m. Ox-ac. Phos. Rhus-t. Sep. STRAM. Zinc.

MOUTH

BAD TASTE—Ang. Ars. Bapt Bry. CALC. Cale-p. Calc-s. Cann-s. Crot-t. Fl-ac. Gels. Graph, Hydr, Kali-bi, Kali-c. Lyc. MERC. Nat-m. NAT-S. Nux-m. NUX-V. Op. Phyt. Podo. Psor, PULS. Sars. Sep. Sil. SULPH. Sulph-ac. Vib. Zinc.

BITTER TASTE—ACON. Alum. Am-m. Arn. Ars. Aur, Bar.c. Bell. BRY. Calc. CARB-V, Carb-s, Card-m.

Cham. CHEL. CHIN. Cocc. COLO. Crot-h. Dig, **Eup-per.** Ferr. Graph. Kali-c. Lach. **Lept.** Lyc. **Merc.** Mur-ac. NAT-M. **NAT-S.** Nux-m. **NUX-V.** Petr. **Phos. PODO. PULS.** Rhus-t. **Sep. SULPH.** Verat.

DRYNESS OF THE—
ACON. Apis. ARS. **Ars-s-f. Bar-c. Bar-m. BELL. Bor. BRY.** Calc. **CANN-I. Canth. CAPS.** Carb-s. **CARB-V.** Caust. **CHAM.** Chel. **CHIN.** Cocc. **CROT-C. CROT-H.** Cupr. Dulc. Ferr. Gels. Graph. **HYOS. IGN. KALI-BI.** Kali-c. **Kali-chl.** Kali-i. Kali-n. **Kali-p. LACH. LAUR.** Lil-t. **LYC.** Mag-m. **MERC.** Mez. **MUR-AC. Naja. Nat-ar. Nat-c. NAT-M. NUX-M. NUX-V.** Op. **Phos-ac. PHOS.** Puls. Rhod.**RHUS-T.** Sars. **SEP. SIL.** Stram. **SULPH. Verat. Verat-v.**

INSIPID TASTE—
Alum. **ANAC.** Ant-t. Ars. **Aur.** Bapt. **Bry.** Caps. **Chin.** Cocc. Colch. Cycl. Dig. Eup-per. **Ferr. Guai. Ip.** Kali-c. Lyc. **MERC.**

Mur-ac. Nat-c. **NAT-M.** Nux-m. Op. petr. **Phos. Psor. PULS.** Sanic. Sep. **Stann.** Staph. **Sulph.** Thuj. Verat. Zinc.

METALLIC TASTE—
Agn. **Am-c.** Arg-n. **Ars.** Bism. **Calc.** Canth. **Cinnb. COCC. Coloc. Cupr.** Ferr-i. Hep. Kali-bi. **Lach.** Lyc. **MERC. Mer-c.** Nat-ar. **NAT-C. Nux-v.** Phyt. **PLB.** Puls. **RHUS-T. SENEG. Sep.** Sil. **Sulph.** Tub. **Zinc.**

OFFENSIVE ODOUR FROM—Agar. **Ambr.** Anac. **ARN. ARS. Ars-i. AUR. BAPT. Bar-c. Bell. Bry.** Calc. Caps. **CARB-AC.** Carb-s. **CARB-V.** Caust. **CHAM. CHEL. Chin.** Cimic. Dulc. **Fl-ac.** Gels. Graph. **Hep.** Hyos. Iod. **Kali-bi.** Kali-c. Kali-i. **Kali-p. KREOS.** Lac-c. **LACH.** Lys. **MERC. MERC-C. Mur-ac. NAT-M.** Nat-s. **NIT-AC.** Nux-m. **Nux-V.** Petr. Phos-ac. **Phyt. PLB. PULS.** Rhus-t. Sep. **Stann. SULPH. Sulph-ac. TUB.** Verb. Zinc.

SALTISH TASTE—Am-c. **Ars.** Ars-i. Bar-c. Bry. **Calc.** Carb-s. **Carb-v.** Carl. Cupr. **Cycl.** Fl-ac. **Graph.** Hyos. Kali-bi. **Kali-chl.** Lach. Mag-m. **MERC. MERC-C.** Nat-c. **NAT-M.** Nit-ac. **Nux-m. Nux-v.** Op. Phos-ac. **Phos. PULS.** Rhus-t. **Sep. sulph.** Tarax. Verat. **Zinc.**

SOUR TASTE—Alum. **Alumn. Ant-c. ARG-N.** Ars. Ars-i. Aur. **Bar-c. CALC.** Calc-s. Carb-s. **Caust.** Cham. **Chin.** Crot-h. Ferr. Graph. **Hep. IGN.** Kali-chl. Kalm. Lach. **LYC. MAG-C.** Mag-m. **MERC.** Mur-ac. **NAT-C.** Nat-m. **NAT-P.** Nit-ac. **Nux-m. NUX-V.** Ox-ac. Petr. Phos-ac. **PHOS. Puls.** Sars. **Sep.** Sil. Stann. **Sulph** Sulph-ac. Tarax. Verat.

SWEETISH TASTE—**Acon.** Alum. Alumn. **Ars.** Aur. Bar-m. **Bell.** Bry. Calc. **Chin.** Coff. **CUPR. DULC.** Ferr. Fl-ac. Hydr-ac. Kali-bi. **Kali-c. Kali-i.** Lach. **LYC.** Mag-c. **Merc.** Mur-ac. Nat-c. Nux-v. Op. **Phos.** Plb. **Podo. PULS. Pyrog.** Sabad.

Sars. Sep. Spong. **STANN. SULPH.** Thuj. zinc.

T R E M B L I N G TONGUE—Agar. **Apis** Arn. Ars. **Aur. Bell. CAMPH.** Canth. Carb-ac. **Crot-h.** Cupr. **GELS. Hell.** Hyos. **IGN. LACH.** Lyc. **MERC.** Mur-ac. Op. Phos-ac. **PLB.** Rhus-t. Sec. Stram. **Tarax.** Vip. zinc.

THROAT

CHOKING—Acon. Apis. Ars. Bapt. **Bell. Cact. Canth.** Carb-v. **CAUST. Cham.** Crot-h. **Cupr. Dig.** Ferr. Fl-ac. **GFLS. Glon.** Graph. Hell. Hep. **HYOS. IGN.** Iod. Ip. Kali-c. Kali-s. **LAC-C. LACH. LAUR.** Lyc. Mag-p. Merc. Mez. **Mosch. NAJA** Nat-m. Nux-v. Phos. **Phyt.** Plat. **PLB.** Puls. Rhod. Sep. **SPONG. Stram. Stry. SULPH.** Tab. Verat. Zinc.

STOMACH

DISTENSION OF THE—Abrot. **Acon. AEth.**

AGAR. All-c. ALOE Alum. **Ant-c.** Ant-t. Apis. **Apoc.** Arg-m. **ARG-N.** Arn. **ARS. ASAF.** Aur. **Bapt.** Bar-c. Bar-m. Berb. Bov. Brom. Bry. Calc. Canth. **CARB-V. Carb-s.** Caust. **Cham. Chel. CHIN.** Cic. Cocc. **COLCH. COLOC.** Con. Croc. Dig. Gamb. **GRAPH.** Hell. **HEP.** Iod. **Jatr.** Kali-bi. **KALI-C.** Kali-p. **LACH. LYC.** Mag-c. Mag-p. **MERC.** Mur-ac. **NAT-C.** Nat-m. **NAT-P. NAT-S. NUX-M. NUX-V. Op.** Petr. **PHOS-AC. PHOS. Podo. PULS. RAPH.** Rhus-t. **Sec. Sep. Sil.** Stann. **Staph. Stram.** Stron-met. **SULPH.** Tab. **TER.** Thuj. **Valer. VERAT. Zinc.**

EASY SATIETY—Am-c. Bry. Caust. **CHIN. Chel.** Dig. **Ferr.** Hydr. **Ign. LYC.** Mag-c. **Nat-m. NUX-M.** Nux-v. Op. Phos. **PLAT.** Podo. Rhod. **Sep.** Sil. **Sulph. Thuj.**

ERUCTATIONS, **AMEL.**—Ant-t. **ARG-N.** Aur. Bar-c. Canth. **Carb-s. CARB-V.** Dig. Dios. Fl-ac. **GRAPH.** Hydr. **IGN. KALI-BI. KALI-C.** Kali-i **Kali-s.** Lac-ac. **Lach. LYC.** Mag-c. Mosch. **Nat-c.** Nit-ac. **NUX-V.** Op. Phos-ac. Phos. **Pic-ac.** Plat. **SANG. Sep. Sil. Sulph.** Tarent. Tereb. Zinc.

FERMENTATION IN THE—Agar. Ambr. Brom. **Bry.** Calc. Carb-an. **CARB-V. CHIN.** Coff. Croc. **Gran.** Hell. **Hep. LYC.** Mag-m. Mur-ac. **Nat-m. NAT-S. Phos.** Plb. Rhus-t. **Sars.** Seneg. Stram. **Sulph.**

AFTER FRUIT– CHIN, GURGLING IN THE**—Agar. ALOE** Arg-n. **Ars.** Bry. Carb-s. **Cocc.** Coloc. **CROT-T. Dros.** Ferr-p. **Gamb.** Graph. Hell. Hyos. Ign. Kali-bi. Lach. **LYC.** Mag-c. Merc. Mur-ac. Nat-c. Nat-m. **Nux-v. OLEAND.** Op. Phos-ac. **Phos. PODO. Psor. PULS. Raph.** Sil. **SULPH.** Thuj. Verb. Zinc.

HEART-BURN—AEsc. **Alum. AMBR. AM-C.** Anac. **Arg-n. Ars.** Berb. **Bry. CALC.**

Carb-an. **CARB-V.** Caust. **Chel. Chin. CIC.** Coff. **CON. CROC.** Dulc. Ferr. **FERR-P.** Fl-ac. **GRAPH.** Hep. Iod. **IRIS. Kali-c. Lach.** Lob. **LYC. MAG-C.** Merc. Nat-m. **NAT-P. NAT-S.** Nux-m. **NUX-V. Phos.** Podo. **PULS. Rob.** Sec. **Sep.** Sil. **SULPH.-AC.** Syph. Thuj. Valer. Verat-v. **Zinc.**

RAVENOUS APPETITE — Alum. **AM-C. ANAC. ARG-M. Ars-i.** Aur. Bar-i. **CALC.** Calc-s. **CANN-I.** Carb-s. **CHIN. CINA.** Con. Ferr. Fl-ac. **GRAPH.** Ign. **IOD.** Kali-n. **Kali-p.** Lac-ac. **LYC.** Mag-m. **Merc. Mur-ac. NAT-M. NUX-V. OLND. PETR.** Phos-ac. **PHOS. PSOR. Puls. SABAD.** Sec. **Sep. SIL.** Spong. **Stann. STAPH. SULPH.** Thuj. **VERAT.** Zinc.

EMACIATION, WITH — Abrot. **CALC. IOD. NAT-M. PETR. Phos.** Psor. **Sulph. TUB.**

SENSITIVE   TO CLOTHING — Apis **ARG-N.**

Benz-ac. **BOV. CALC. Carb-v.** Caust. Chin. Coff. **CROT-C. Crot-h.** Eup-per. **Graph. HEP. Kreos. Lac-c. LACH. LYC.** Merc-c. Nat-s. **NUX-V.** Puls. Raph. **Sars. Sep. Spong. stann.** Sulph.

AFTER   EATING— **Graph. LYC.** Nux-v.

THIRST—Acet-ac. Ant-c. **ACON.** Arg-n. **ARS.** Bell. **BRY. CALC. Calc-s. Caust. Cham. Chin.** Crot-h. **DIG. EUP-PER. Graph. HELL.** Hep. **Iod. Kali-br. Kali-p. Kreos.** Lyc. **MERC-C. NAT-M. Nat-s.** Nux-v. Op. Petr. Podo. Rhus-t. **Rob.** Sep. **SIL. STRAM. SULPH.** Sulph-ac. **VERAT.** Zinc.

THIRSTLESSNESS — Ant-c. **ANT-T. APIS** Arg-n. Bov. Caps. **CHIN. COLCH.** Con. **CYCL.** Ferr. **GELS. HELL.** Hydr-ac. **Ip. Kali-c. Lyc. MENY.** Nat-c. **NUX-M.** Nux-v. Petr. **PHOS-AC. PULS. SABAD.** Sep. Sulph. Thuj. Valer. Verat.

WANTING, APPETITE

— Agar. ANT-C. ARS. ASAR.
Bapt. Bar-c. Bor. Bry. Cact.
CALC. Carb-an. Carb-v.
CHAM. Chel. CHIN. Cina.
COCC. Con. CYCL. Dig.
FERR. Fl-ac. Graph. Hydr. Ip.
KALI-BI. Kali-s. LYC. Mag-c.
Merc. NAT-M. Nux-m. NUX-
V. Op. Petr. Phos-ac. PHOS. Plb.
Podo. Psor. PULS. Rhus-t. Sang.
SEP. SIL. Stann. SULPH.
Sulph-ac.Syph. Tereb. Thuj.
Verat.

WATER-BRASH —

Alumn. Am-c. am-m. Ant-t.
Apis. ARS. BAR-C. Bism. BRY.
CALC. Calc-p. Carb-an. CARB-
V. Chin. Cocc. Dig. Ferr. Graph.
Hep. Ip. Kali-bi. KALI-C. Lach.
LYC. Mag-m. Merc. MEZ. Nat-
c. Nat-m. Nit-ac. Nux-v. Par.
PETR. PHOS. Podo. PULS.
Rhus-t. SABAD. SANG. Sep.
SIL. STAPH. SULPH.
SULPH. Sulph-ac. Thuj. Verat.
Zinc.

RECTUM

CONSTIPATION —

Abr. AESC. Aloe. ALUM.
ALUMN. Anac. ANT-C. Apis.
Ars. AUR. BAR-C. BAR-M.
BRY. Calc. Carb-s. Carb-v.
CAUST. Chel. Chin. Clem.
Cocc. Coff. Coll. Coloc. CON.
Dios. Ferr. GRAPH. HEP. HYDR.
Ign. KALI-M. LAC-D. Lach.
LYC. MAG-M. MAG-S.
MERC. MEZ. Mur-ac. NAT-
M. NIT-AC. Nux-m. NUX-V.
Enan.OP. Phos. PLAT. PLB.
Puls. Ruta SANIC. SEL. SEP.
SIL. Staph. Stram. STRY.
SULPH. Thuj. VERAT.
ZINC.

DIARRHEA —Agar.

ALOE ANT-C. Ant-t. Apis.
ARG-N. ARS. Bapt. Bar-c. Bry.
CALC. CALC-P. Canth.
CARB-V. Cham. CHIN. Coloc.
Corn. CROT-T. Dios. DULC.
FERR. Ferr-ar. Ferr-i. FERR-
P. Fl-ac. GAMB. Hell. Hep.
Iod. IP. IRIS. Kali-bi. KALI-
P. Lept. Lyc. Merc. Merc-c. Nat-

m. NAT-S. NIT-AC. Nux-m. NUX-V. Petr. PHOS-AC. PHOS. Plb. PODO. Psor. Puls. Rheum. SEC. Sep. SIL. SULPH. THUJ. Valer. VERAT Zing.

DYSENTERY—Acon. ALOE Arg-n. **Arn. ARS. BAPT.** Bell. Bry. CANTH. Caps. Carb-v. COLCH. COLOC. Dulc. HAM. IP. Kali-bi. KALI-M. Lach. Mag-c. Mag-p. MERC. MERC-C. Nit-ac. NUX-V. PHOS. Puls. RHUS-T. SULPH. Throm. Verat.

FLATUS, AMEL.—Aloe **Arg-n.** Aur. Bry. calc-p **Carb-s. CARB-V.** Cham. **Chin. Cocc.** Colch. **Coloc.** Graph. Ign. Kali-c. Lach. **LYC.** Mez. **NAT-S.** Nux-m. **NUX-V.** Phos-ac. **Phos. Plb. PULS.** Rhod. **SANG. SULPH.** Thuj. **Verat.** Zinc.

HEMORRHOIDS IN THE —AEsc. Ant-c. ARS. Bell. Calc-p. **CAPS. CARB-V. Caust.** COLL. Dios. Ferr. **Fl-ac.** GRAPH. HAM. Hep. **Hydr.**

IGN. Kali-ar. **Kali-bi.** Kali-c. Kali-s. **Mag-m. Merc. MUR-AC. Nat-m. NIT-AC.** Podo. **Puls.** Ruta **SEP.** Sil. Staph. SULPH. THUJ. Zinc.

PULSATION   IN THE—ALOE Alum. Alumn. Am-m. Apis. **Berb.** Calc-p. **Caps.** Caust Grat. **Ham. LACH.** Meli. **NAT-M.** Rhod. Seneg. **SULPH.**

BLADDER

BALL   IN   THE, SENSATION OF A—Crot-h. **Lach.** Naja

DYSURIA – ACON. **Agar. Alum. APIS ARG-N.** Arn. **Ars. BELL. Berb. Calc-p.** Camph. **CANN-S. CANTH. Caps. Chin. CLEM.** Con. **COP.** Cupr. **DIG.** Dulc. Eup-per. **Gels. Hep.** Kali-c. **LIL-T. LYC.** Merc. **MERC-C.** Nat-m. Nit-ac. **NUX-V. OP. PAREIR. Petros. Plb. PULS.** Rhus-t. Senec. **SEP.** Sil. Stram.**SULPH.** Tarent. **TEREB. Thuj.** Uva. Verat. Zinc.

FEEBLE STREAM—
ALUM. Apis ARG-N. Bell.
Berb. Calc-p. Camph. Cann-I.
Caust. CLEM. Dig. Gels. Hell.
HEP. Kali-bi. Kali-c. Kali-p.
Kreos. Laur. Lyc. Med. MERC.
MERC-C. Mur-ac. Nat-m. Nit-
ac. OP. Petr. Phos-ac. Prun. Puls.
SARS. Sep. Stram. SULPH.
Thuj. Zinc.

FULNESS, SENSATION
OF, IN THE—Apis Arg-n. Arn.
Ars. Bell. Calad. CHIM. Cub.
DIG. EQUIS. Gels. Hell. Kali-
i. Lyc. Med. Merc. Merc-c.
NUX-V. OP. Puls. Ruta Sep.
Staph. Stram. Sulph. Thuj.
Zinc.

MUST HASTEN TO
URINATE OR URINE WILL
ESCAPE—Agar. Aloe. Arg-n.
ARN. Bar-c. Bell. Bry. Camph.
CANTH. CLEM. Coc-c. Dulc.
Ferr-p. Hyos. KREOS. Merc.
NUX-V. Petros. Phos. Plb.
PULS. SEP. Squil. Staph. Stram.
SULPH. Thuj. Verat. Zinc.

KIDNEYS

PULSATION IN
THE— Act-s. Berb. Bufo.
Canth. Chel. Kali-i. Med. Pic-ac.
Sabin. Sulph.

SUPPRESSION OF
URINE—Acon. APIS Arn.
ARS. Bell. Camph. CANTH.
Carb-ac. CARB-V. Cic. Colch.
Crot-h. Cupr. Dig. Erig. Hell.
HYOS. Kali-bi. LACH. LAUR.
LYC. Merc-c. OP. Phos. Plb.
SEC. Sil. STRAM. Sulph.
Tarent. Tereb. Urt-u. VERAT.
Zinc.

URINE

ALBUMINOUS
URINE—Ant-t. APIS Arg-n.
ARS. Aur. AUR-M. Aur-m-n.
Calc. CALC-AR. Cann-s.
CANTH. Colch. Dig. Ferr-p.
Gels. Glon. Hell. Iod. KALI-
C. Lac-d. Lach. LYC. Merc.
MARC-C. Nat-ar. NAT-C.
Nat-m. PHOS-AC. PHOS.
Rhus-t. Sulph. TEREB. Uran.
Zinc.

BLACK URINE–Ars. Canth. **CARB-AC. COLCH.** Dig. Hell. Kali-c. Kali-chl. **LACH. Merc-c. Nat-m.** Pareir. **Phos.** Sec. **TEREB.** Verat.

BROWN URINE – Acon. Ambr. **ARN. ARS.** Bell. **BENZ-AC. BRY.** Carb-ac. **CHEL.** Colch. Dig. Hell. **Kreos.** Lach. Lyc. Merc. **MER-C. Nit-ac.** Phos. **Puls.** Stram. Sulph. Valer. Zinc.

GREENISH URINE – Ars. Aur. Bapt. Berb. **CAMPH.** Chel. **Chin.** Chim. **Colch.** Cop. Crot-h. Dig. Kali-c. **Mag-c MERC-C. Nit-ac.** Phos. Rheum. Rhod. **Ruta.** Sulph. Uran. Verat.

PALE URINE – Alum. Am-c. Arg-m. Ars. Bell. Bry. **Cann-I.** Carb-v. **Clem.** Colch. **CON.** Dig. Ferr. **GELS.** Hep. **Ign. KALI-N.** Kreos. **Lac d. LED. Lyc.** Mag-c. **MERC-C. NAT-M. Nat-s.** Nux-v. **PHOS-AC.** Phos. Plan. Rhod. **SARS.** Staph. Stram. Sulph. Verat.

RED URINE – Acon. **Apis.** Bapt. **BELL. BENZ-AC.** Berb. **BRY.** Cact. Camph. **CANTH.** Carb-v. **Chel.** Colch. Dulc. Ferr-p. **Iod. Kali-bi. LYC.** Merc. Mur-ac. Plat. Puls. **Sel. SEP. STRAM, Sulph. Tereb.** Thuj. Zinc.

SUGAR IN THE URINE – Acet-ac. **ARG-M. Ars.** Benz-ac. **BOV.** Calc. Calc-p. **Carb-ac.** Carb-v. **Chel.** Chin. **Colch.** Elaps. **Ferr-m. HELON.** Hep. Iris. **KALI-P.** Kreos. **Lac d. Lach. LYC.** Med. **Merc. Nat-s.** Nit-ac. Op. **PHOS-AC. PHOS. Pic-ac. PLB.** Sil. **Sulph. TARENT. TEREB.** Thuj. **URAN. ZINC.**

YELLOW URINE – **Agar. Aloe.** Am-m. Ant-c. Ars. **AUR.** Bar-m **Bell.** Berb. **Cann-s.** Cham. **CHEL.** Chin. Colch. Crot-t. **Daph. Hyos.** Iod. **LACH.** Mag-m. Nat-c. Nit-ac. Plb. **SEP.** Verat.

MALE SEXUAL ORGANS

COITION, AVERSION TO–Agar. **Agn. Cann-s. GRAPH.** Kali-c. **LYC.** Nat-m. Petr. Phos. **Psor. Sulph.**

COLDNESS OF PENIS–Agar. **AGN.** Bar-c Caps. Dios. Ind. **LYC.** Merc. **ONOS. SULPH.**

HYDROCELE –APIS. Arn. Calc. **Dig.** Fl-ac. **GRAPH.** HEP. **IOD.** Lyss. **Merc.** Nat-m. Nux-v. **Phos. Psor. PULS. RHOD.** Sel. **SIL.** Spong. **SULPH.** Sulph-ac.

" BRUISE, CAUSED BY A–Arn.

" GONORRHEAL OR CHITIS, AFTER–Phos.

"   HERPETIC ERUPTION – WITH– GRAPH.

INCOMPLETE ERE-CTION –Agar. **AGN. Ars. CALAD. Camph.** Cob. **CON.** Form. **GRAPH.** Hep. Lach. **LYC.** Merc.**Nat-c. Nat-m.** Nuph. **NUX-V.** Petr. **Phos-ac. PHOS. SEL.** SEP. Sil. **SULPH.**

SEXUAL PASSION, DIMINISHED – Agar. **AGN.** Alum. Aur. **BAR-C.** Calc-p. Clem. **DIOS.** Ferr. **GRAPH.** Hep. Ign. Kali-c. Kali-i **Kali-p. LYC.** Mag-c. **Mur-ac. Nat-m. Nit-ac.** Nuph. **Op. Phos-ac. Psor.** Rhod. Sel. **Sep. SIL. STAPH. Sulph.** Ther.

SEXUAL PASSION, INCREASED – **Agar. Am-c. Anac. ANAN.** Ant-c. **AUR.** Bar-c. **BAR-M.** Brom. **Bufo CALC.** Calc-p. **CAMPH. CANN-I. CANN-S. CANTH.** Cast. Chin. Cocc. Coff. Con. Dios. Ferr. **Gels. Graph.** Hyos. **Ign.** Kali-p. Lach. **LYC. LYSS.** Merc. Mosch. nat-c. **Nat-m.** Nit-ac. **NUX-V. Op. Phos-ac. PHOS. PIC-AC. PLAT.** Plb. **Psor. PULS.** Sep. Sil. Stann. **Staph. Stram. Sulph.** Tarent. Thuj. **TUB.** Ust. Verat. **ZINC.**

FEMALE SEXUAL ORGANS

COITION, AVERSION

TO—Agn. Am-c. Bov. Cann-s. Caust. Clem. Ferr-p. **Graph.** Ign. **Kali-br.** Kali-p. **Lach.** Lyc. **Med. NAT-M.** Op. Petr. **Phos. Plb. Psor.** Rhod. **SEP.** Stann. sulph. Thuj.

DESIRE. INCREASED

–Ant-c. **APIS** Ars. Aur. Bar-m. **Bell.** Calad. **CALC. CALC-P. CAMPH.** Cann-I. **CANTH.** Carb-v. **Coff. CON.** Dulc. **FL-AC.** Gels. **GRAT. HYOS.** Ign. **Kali-br. KALI-P.** Kreos. Lac-c. **LACH. LIL-T.** Lyc. Merc. **Mosch. MUREX.** Nat-c. Nat-m. **NUX-V.** Op. Orig. **PHOS. PIC-AC. PLAT PULS.** Sabin. Sil. **Stann. Staph.** Stram Tarent. Thuj. **VERAT.** Zinc.

ENJOYMENT ABSENT

– Alum. **Berb. Brom.** Calc. Cann-s. **CAUST. FERR.** Ferr-m **GRAPH.** Kali-br. Lyss. **Med. Nat-m.** Onos. **Phos.** Plat. Puls. **SEP.**

LEUCORRHEA – Alet.

ALUM. Am-c. Am-m. **Arg-n. ARS. Ars-i. Aur-m.** Bar-c. **BOR.** Bov. **CALC.** Calc-p. **Calc-s. CAUST.** Cocc. Ferr. Gels. Graph. Hep. **IOD.** Kali-ar. **KALI-BI. KALI-C.** Kali-chl. Kali-i. Kali-p. Kali-s. **KREOS.** Lac-c. **Lach. Lyc.** Mag-m. **MED. MERC.** Merc-c. Mur-ac. Nat-c. **NAT-M.** Nat-s. **NIT-AC.** Nux-m. Orig. Petr. **Phos-ac. PLAT.** Psor. **PULS. SEP.** Sil. **STANN. SULPH. SULPH-AC. SYPH. Thuj.** Zinc.

METRORRHAGIA–

Acon. Arn. Ars. **Bell. Both.** Bry. **Calc.** Canth. Carb-v. **CHIN.** Colch. Coloc. **CROC. CROT-H.** ERIG. **FERR.** Ferr-p. **HAM.** Hyos. Iod. **IP.** Kali-c. **KALI-FCY.** Kreos. **LACH.** Lyc. **MILL. MUREX.** Nat-c. **NIT-AC.** Nux-m. **NUX-V. PHOS. PLAT. PSOR. PULS. Rat. SABIN. SEC.** Senec. **Sep.** Sil. **SULPH.** Tarent **TRIL.** Zinc. **UST.** Verat. Zinc.

LARYNX AND TRACHEA

HOARSENESS

ACON. ALL-C. Alum. Ambr. Am-c. Am-m. Ant-t. ARG-M. ARG-N. Ars. ARUM-T. Bar-c. Bell. BROM. Bry. CALC. Calc-s. Canth. Caps. CARB-V. CAUST. Cham. Chlor. Cupr. DROS. Dulc. Euphr. Ferr-p. Gels. HEP. Hyos. IOD. KALI-BI. Kali-c. Kali-chl. Kali-p. Kali-s. LACH. Laur. Lyc. Mag-m. MANG. MERC. NAJA NAT-M. Nit-ac. Nux-v. Op. Petr. PHOS. Phyt. Puls. Rhus-t. SEL. Sep. SPONG. STANN. STRAM. Sulph. TELL. Thuj. Verat. Zinc. ZING.

RATTLING, IN THE LARYNX

– Am-c. ANT-T. Bar-c. Carb-v. Caust. Euphr. Ferr-p. HEP. HYOS. IP. Kali-c. Kali-s. Laur. Merc. Nat-m. Nit-ac. Op. Puls. Samb. Sep. Sulph.

TICKLING, IN THE TRACHEA

– Acon. Agar. Bell. Bry. Calc. Caps. Carb-s. Carb-v. Cham. Con. Dulc. Euphr. Ferr. Hyos. Iod. Kali-bi. KALI-C. Kalm. Lach. Med. Nat-s. Nux-v. PHOS-AC. Phos. Psor. PULS. RHUS-T. RUMEX. SANG. Seneg. Sep. Sil. Spong. STANN. Stict. Still. Sulph. Thuj. Verat. Zinc.

RESPIRATION

ASTHMATIC

– Acon. AMBR. Am-c. ANT-T. Apis. ARG-N. ARS. Ars-i. Asaf. Aur. Bar-c. Bell. BLATTA-A. Bov. Brom. Bry. Cact. Calc. Cann-s. Caps. CARB-V. Chin. Chlor. CUPR. Dig. Dulc. Ferr. FERR-P. Graph. Hep. Ign. IP. Kali-ar. Kali-br. KALI-C. Kali-chl. Kali-i. KALI-N. KALI-P. Kali-s. Lach. Led. LOB. Lycl. Med. Meph. Mosch. Naja NAT-S. NUX-V. Op. PHOS. PULS. Ruta SAMB. Sang. Seneg. Sep. SIL. SPONG. Stann. Stram. SULPH. Sulph-ac. Thuj. Verat. Zinc.

SNORING

–Arn. Ars. Brom. Camph. Cham. Chin.

Cic. Cupr. **Dros.** Glon. **Hep. Hyos. Ign.** Kali-bi. **LAC-C. Lach. Laur.** Lyc. Mur.ac. Nit-ac. **Nux v. OP.** Petr. **Rhus-t.** Samb. Sil. Stann. **Stram. Sulph.**

STERTOROUS

Acon. Am-c. Ant-t. Apis. **Ars.** Bell. **Camph.** Carb-ac. Chin. Cupr,**Gels. Glon.** Hydr-ac. Kali-bi. **Lach. Laur.** Lyc. Nit-ac. Nux m. **Nux v. OP.** Phos. **Spong. Stram.** Tab.

COUGH

COUGH, BETTER FROM EXPECTORATION –

Ail. Alum. Alumn. Bell. **Calc.** Carb-an. Caust. **Guai. Hep. Iod. Ip.** Kali-n. Kreos. **LACH.** Lob. Meli. Mez. **Phos.** Phyt. **Sang.** Sep. Sulph. Zinc.

DISRESSING – Arum-t. Brom. **CAUST.** Lach. Lyc. Nit-ac. **NUX V.** Sang. **Seneg.** Sep. Squil. Stann.

RATTLING – ANT-T. Arg-m. **Arg-n.** Bar-c. Bell. **Brom.** Bry. Cact. **Calc.** Calc-s. Carb-an. Carb-v. **CAUST.** Cham. **Chel. Coc-c.** Ferr. **Hep.** Hydr.Iod. **IP. Kali-bi. kali-chl.** Kali-p. **KALI-S. Lach.** Lyc. Merc. Nat-m. **Nat-s. Nux v. Op. PHOS. Puls.** Samb. **SEP.** Sil. **Squil. Stann. Sulph.** Verat.

CHEST

ANXIETY, IN REGION OF HEART –

ACON. Ambr. **Aml-ns. Ant-t. ARG-N. ARS. AUR.** Bell. **Brom. CACT.** Calc. Camph. **CARB-V. Cinch.** Coff. Cupr. Dig. Ferr. **FERR-P. Gels. Glon. HYDR-AC. IGN.** Iod. **Ip. KALM.** Lach. Lyc. **Meny.** Merc. **Naja Nux-v.** Op. **PHOS.** Plb. **Plat.** Prun. Psor. **Puls.** Rhus-t. Spig. Spong. **Tab.** Tarent. **THER. Verat.** Viol-t. Vip.

CARDIAC DILA-TATION – Alum. **AM-C.** Ant-t. Apis **ARS.** Aur. **CACT.** Coff. Cupr. **Hydr-ac. Iod. Kali-i. LACH. Laur.** Lil-t. **Lyc.** Lycps.

NAJA. **Nat-m.** Nux-v. Phos-ac. **PHOS.** Plb. **Psor.** Puls. Tab. Verat.

CARDIAC HYPER-TROPHY – ACON. **Aml-ns.** ARN. **Ars.** Aspar. AUR. **AUR-I.** Aur-m. Brom. CACT. Dig. Ferr. Glon. Graph. Hep. **Iber. Iod.** Kali-bi. **KALI-C. KALM. Lach. LITH. Lyc.** Lycps. **Naja. Nat-m.** Nux-v. PHOS. Plb. Puls. Rhus-t. Spig. SPONG. Staph.

" WITH NUMBNESS AND TINGLING OF LEFT ARM AND FINGERS– ACON. RHUS-T.

COLDNESS IN THE – ACON. **Am-m.** Arg-m. **Ars.** Bell. **Bor.** Bry. CACT. **Camph.** Canth. **CAPS.** Cham. Con. Dig. Dulc. EUP-PER. EUP-PUR. Ferr. **Gels.** Ham. Hyos. Ign. Kali-c. Lac-d. **LACH.** Led. Lil-t. **Meny.** Mez. NAT-M. NAT-S. Nit-ac. **Nux-v.** Phos. PULS. Rhus-t. **Sil.** Stann. Stry. SULPH. VERAT.

CONSTRICTION, TENSION, TIGHTNESS IN THE – ACON. Agar. Am-c. Ant-t. Apis. Arg-n. **ARS. AUR.** Bapt. **BELL.** Bor. **BROM. BRY. CACT. Calc.** Calc-p. Carb-s. **CARB-V. CAUST. Chel.** Chlor. Cocc. **CON.** Crot-c. **Cupr.** DIG. Dros. Ferr. **FERR-P.** Glon. **Graph.** Hyos. **IGN.** Ip. Kali-bi. **KALI-C.** Kali-p. **LACH.** Mag-p. Merc. **Naja.** Nat-c. **Nat-m.** Nit-ac. Nux-m. **Nux-v.** Op. **PHOS.** Plat. **Puls.** Rhus-t. **SENEG.** Sep. **SIL. Spig.** Spong. Squil. **STANN.** Stram. Sulph. Tab. Thuj. **VERAT.**

PALPITATION— ACON. **Agar.** Ambr. Am-c. **AML-NS.** Apis **ARG-N. ARS. Ars-i.** AUR. **Aur-m.** Bar-c. Bell. Brom-Bry. **CACT. CALC.** Calc-p. Camph. Cann-I. Carb-v. **CHIN. Colch. Con.** Cupr. **DIG.** Ferr. **FERR-P. Gels. GLON.** Hydr-ac. **IOD. KALI-P. KALM.** LACH. Led. Lob. **LYC.** Lycps. Mag-m. **Merc. Mosch.** NAJA. Nat-ar. Nat-c.

NAT-M. Nat-p. **Nux-m.** **NUX-V.** Phos-ac. **PHOS. Puls.** Rhus-t. Sep. **SPIG. Spong.** Staph. **SULPH. TAB. THUJ. VERAT.**

WEAKNESS IN THE –
Aesc. **Agar. ARS.** Bar-c. **Brach. CALC.** Carb-v. Casc. **Cic. Eupper. Gels. GRAPH.** Hydr. Kali-p. Lach. Lyss. Med. **Murex.** **NAT-M. NUX-V.** Ox-ac. **Petr. PHOS-AC. Phos.** Pic-ac. Puls. Rhus-t. **SEL. SEP.** Sil. **SULPH.** Verat-v. **ZINC.**

EXTREMITIES

BURNING, IN THE PALMS – Aesc. Apis. **Ars. CALC. Calc-s. Canth. Carb-v.** Fl-ac. **Graph. LACH.** Lachn. **Lyc. Med.** Merc. Mur-ac. **Nat-c.** Nat-m. Petr. **PHOS.** Rhus-t. **Sang.** Sec. **Sep. STANN. SULPH.** Upa.

BURNING, IN THE SOLES – Aesc. Alum. **Ambr.** Anac. **Ars.** Aur-m. Bell. **CALC. Calc-s. Canth.** Carb-s. **Carb-v.**

Caust. Cham. Cocc. Cupr. Dulc. Fl-ac. **Graph. Kali-p. KALI-S. LACH.** Lachn. **LYC. Mag-m. Manc.** Mang. **MED.** Merc. **Nat-c NAT-S.** Nux-v. Phos-ac. **PHOS.** Plb. **Puls. Sec. SEP.** Sil. Stann. **SULPH. Sulph-i.** Tab. Zinc.

FORMICATION IN THE –**ACON. Agar.** Alum. **Arg-n.** Bar-c. **Camph.** Caust. Hep. **Ign.** Kali-p. lach. **Laur. LYC.** Mez. **Nux-v. PHOS-AC. Phos.** Plb. Puls. Rhod. **Rhus-t.** Sabad. **SEC.** Stram. **Stry. TARENT.** Verat. **Zinc.**

IN-CO ORDINATION IN THE – Agar. **ALUM.** Arg-n. Bell. **Calc.** Carb-s. Caust. Chlor. Coca.**Cocc. CON. Cupr. Gels.** Merc. **Onos. Phos-ac. Phos.** Plb. Sec. Stram. **Sulph.** Tab. **Zinc.**

WEAKNESS IN THE – Agar. **Alum.** Anac. **Arg-m. ARG-N. ARS.** Bar-m. **Bry. CALC.** Calc-p. **CAUST.** Cic. **Cocc. CON.** Cupr. Dulc.

FERR. Ferr-m. GELS. Graph.
Hep. Iod. Kali-bi. KALI-BR.
KALI-C. KALI-P. Kali-s. Kalm.
Lach. LYC. MERC. Nat-c.
Nat-m. NIT-AC. NUX-V.
Op. Petr. Phos-ac. Phos. PIC-
AC. PLB. Psor. Puls. RHUS-T.
Sec. SIL. Stann. STAPH. Sulph.
Tarent. Thuj. Zinc.

SLEEP

DISTURBED – Acon.
Apis. Arn. ARS. Bar-c. BELL.
Cact. Calc-p. Cupr-ar. Dig.
Dulc. Form. GRAPH. Hyos.
Kali-bi. Kali-i. Kali-p. Laur. OP.
Phys. Plb. Puls. Sep. SULPH.
Tab. Vesp.

SLEEPLESSNESS –
Acon. Agar. Aloe. Apis. ARG-
N. Arn. ARS. Ars-i. Aur. Bapt.
BELL. Bor. Bry. CACT. CALC.
Calc-p. Camph. Canth. Carb-v.
CHAM. Chin. cio-v. COFF.
Cycl. Fl-ac. Gels. Glon. Hep.
HYOS. Ign. Kali-br. KALI-C.
KALI-P. Kreos. LACH. Lyc.
MERC. Merc-c. Nat-m. Nat-s.

Nat-s. NUX-V. OP. Plb.
PULS. RHUS-T. Sel. SEP. SIL.
Stram. Staph. SULPH. Syph.
Tab. Tarent. THUJ. VALER.
Verat. Zinc.

PERSPIRATION

COLD – Agar. AM-C.
Anac. ANT-T. Arn. ARS. Bar-c.
CALC. CAMPH. Carb-s.
CARB-V. Chin. Chinin-ars.
COCC. Crot-h. Dros. Elaps.
FERR. Gels. HEP. Hyos. IP.
Lach. Lob. LYC. Merc. MERC-
C. Mez. Mur-ac. Nat-c. Nux-v.
Petr. Phos. Psor. Puls. Ruta SEC.
SEP. Spig. Staph. Sulph. TAB.
Thuj. Tub. VERAT. VERAT-V.

HOT–ACON. Aesc.
BELL. Bry. Calc. Carb-v.
CHAM. Chel. Chin. Cocc.
CON. Dig. IGN. IP. Merc-i-r.
Nat-c. NUX-V. OP Phos.
PSOR. Puls. Pyrog. Sabad. SEP.
Sil. Stann. Staph. STRAM.
Sulph. Thuj. Verat.

PROFUSE – Aml-ns.
ANT-T. Arg-n. ARS. Aur-m.

AUR-M-N. Bapt. Bar-c. BELL.
BRY. Cact. Camph. Caps. Carb-
an. Carb-s. CARB-V. Caust.
Cedr. CHIN. Chinin-ar.
CHININ-S. Cist. Colch. Cupr.
Dig. Eup-per. FERR. Ferr-ar.
Ferr-p. Gels. HEP. Ip. Kali-ar.
Kali-bi. KALI-C. KALI-P. Lac-
ac. Lach. LYC. Mag-c. MERC.
Mez. Nat-c. NAT-M. Nit-ac.
Nux-v. Petr. PHOS-AC. Phos.
Psor. Puls. Rhus-t. Sabad. Samb.
Sec. Sel. Sep. Sil. spong. Stram.
Sulph. Tarax. Thuj. Tub. Valer.
Verat. Zinc.

SYMPTOMS, AGRAVATE
WHILE SWEATING – Ant-t.
Ars. Calc. Caust. Cham. Chin.
Croc. Eup-per. Ferr. FORM Ign.
Ip. Lyc. Merc. Nat-c. Nux-v. Op.
Phos. Puls. Psor. Rhus-t. Sep.
Spong. Stram. Sulph. Verat.

  "   AMELIORATE
WHILE SWEATING – Acon.
Aesc. Aeth. Apis. Ars. Bapt. Bell.
Bov. Bry. Calad. Camph. Canth.
Cham. Chin-s. Cimex. CUPR.
Eup-per. Gels. Lyc. Nat-m. Psor.
Rhus-t. Samb. Sec. Stron-met.
Thuj. Verat.

VI. Therapeutics

1. **Acetanilidum**—It depresses heart, respiration and blood pressure; lowers temperature. **Enlarged sensation in the head. Fainting. Albuminuria, with edema of the feet and ankles.** Pulse weak and irregular.

   Potency —Low potencies, preferably the 3rd.

2. **Aceticum ac.** — Great debility. Frequent fainting, dyspnea and cardiac weakness. Blood rushes to head. Temporal vessls distended. Cheeks hot and flushed. **Intense burning thirst. Vomits after every kind of food. Sour belching and vomiting.** Tympanitic abdomen. Passes large quantities of pale urine. Cough, worse when inhaling. Edema of the feet and legs. Profuse cold sweat.

   Potency —3rd to 30th.

3. **Aconitum nap.**—Dry heat and red face. Thirsty and restless. Chilliness and formication down back. **Formication and numbness.**

Sleeplessness, with tossing about. Bursting headache. As if brain were moved by boiling water. Vertigo, worse on rising (*Nux vom.; Op.*). Pulse full and bounding, almost incompressible. Fears death, but believes that he will soon die. Pains are intolerable; they drive him crazy. Bitter taste of everything except water. Burning from stomach to esophagus.

Potency —3rd to 30th.

4. **Adonis ver.**—Heavy weight in the stomach. Scanty and albuminous urine. Frequent desire to take a long breath (Ignatia, Lachesis, Phosphorus). Feeling of weight on the chest. It is useful in lowering arterial pressure. Pulse rapid and irregular. Cardiac asthma. Marked venous engorgement. Precordial pain, palpitation and dyspnea. Spine stiff and aching.

    Potency—Tinct. (5 to 10 drops), 3rd to 30th.

5. **Adrenalinum**—Useful in Arteriosclerosis and blood pressure. Vertigo, nausea and vomiting are prominent. Is invaluable in checking capillary hemorrhages from almoset all parts. Despondency, aversion to mental work, cannot concentrate. Congestion of brain with fulness in

head. Headache with aching in eyeballs, better by pressure on eyes and walking in open air. Flushes of heat over head and face.

Potency—Ix to 6x.

6. **Agaricus musc.**—**Jerking, twitching, trembling** and **itching** are strong indications. Aversion to work. Indifference. **Headache, with nose-bleed or thick mucous discharge. Double vision** (*Gelsemium*). **Laboured, oppressed breathing. Cough ends in a sneeze. Pulse irregular and intermittent.** Redness of the face supervene with palpitation. Cough with expectoration of little balls of mucus. Gastric disturbance with sharp pain in the right hypochondrium.

Potency —3rd to 30th and 200th.

7. **Alumen**—Great weakness of the chest. Asthma of old people. Copious, ropy expectoration in the morning. **Hemoptysis. Palpitation from lying down on the right hand side. Obstinate constipation. No desire for stool for days together. Marble-like masses pass, till the rectum feels loaded.** Vertigo. Mental paresis.

Dysphagia, especially to liquids. Every cold settles in throat.

Potency — 1st to 30th and higher.

8. **Ambra gris.**—Desires to be alone. Loathing of life. Patient weakened by age and overwork. Slow comprehension. **Rush of blood to head. Epistaxis, especially in the morning. Eructations with violent, convulsive cough.** Sensation of coldness in the abdomen. Urine turbid, even during emission, forming a brown sediment. Palpitation, with pressure in the chest as from a lump lodged there.

Potency — 3rd to 30th and higher.

9. **Ammoniacum gum.**—Stars and fiery points float before the eyes. Dim vision. Easily fatigued from reading. **Chronic bronchial catarrh. Tough and hard mucus, is dislodged with great difficulty.** Heart beats stronger, extends to the pit of the stomach. Throat feels dry. Difficult breathing.

Potency —Lower trits. to 30th.

10. **Ammonium carb.**—Shocks through the head. Pulsating pain in the forehead; better from hard

pressure. Aversion to light. Forgetfulness. Ill-humoured. **Stoppage of nostrils at night, with long continued coryza. Epistaxis in morning, on washing and after eating.** Nose congested. Great appetite, but easily satisfied. Stools, difficult, hard and knotty. Bloody piles, worse during menses. White, sandy, bloody, copious, turbid or fetid urine. Chest feels tired. Slow, labored, stertorous breathing.

Potency —6th. to 200th.

11.   **Amylenum nit.**—Palpitation of the heart and similar conditions are readily cured by it, especially the flushings and other discomforts at climacteric. **Hiccough and yawning. Surging of blood to the head and face. Sense of constriction in the throat. Collar seems too tight. Dyspnea and asthmatic feelings. Great oppression and fulness of chest. Precordial anxiety. Tumultuous action of the heart. Much flushing of** heat; sometimes followed by cold and clammy skin and profuse sweat. Throbbing throughout the whole body. Constant stretching for hours.

Potency —3rd to 30th.

12.   **Angustura vera**—Pain in the knees. Cracking in the joints. Arms feel tired and heavy. **Drawing in the nape of the neck. Headache, with heat of face. Acute pain in cheeks. Drawing in facial muscles. Cramp-like pain on the zygomatic arch.** Irresistible desire for coffee. Atonic dyspepsia. Belching with cough. Bitter taste in the mouth. Tenesmus with soft stool. Burning in the anus.

Potency —6th to 200th.

13.   **Antimonium crud.**—Much concerned about his fate. **Cross and contradictive; whatever is done, fails to give him satisfaction. Sulky, does not wish to speak. Peevish. Vexed without cause. Heaviness in the forehead, with vertigo. Tongue coated thick white, as if white-washed.** Loss of appetite. Desire for acids and pickles. Eructation tasting of the ingesta. Heartburn, nausea and vomiting. Alternate diarrhea and constipation. Cough, worse when coming in a warm room.

Potency —3rd to 30th.

14.   **Antipyrinum**—Epileptiform   seizures. Contractures. Trembling and cramps. **Genral**

prostration. Oppression and dyspnea. Faintness, with sensation of stoppage of heart. **Cheyne-stokes respiration.** Rapid, weak and irregular pulse. Throbbing throughout the whole body. Edema and puffiness of the face. Urine diminished.

Ponency —Low decimals.

15. **Apis mell.**— Lids swollen, red, edematous. Pale, waxy or edematous countenance. **Thirstlessness.** Vomiting of food. Craving for milk. **Urine suppressed; loaded with casts; scanty and high-colored.** Constipation. Feels, as if something would break on straining. hemorrhoids, with stinging pains. Feels, as if he would not be able to draw another breath. Sudden puffing up of the whole body.

Potency —1st to 30th.

16. **Argentum nit.**—Headache with coldness and trembling. Brain-fag, with general debility and trembling. Vertigo, with buzzing in the ears. **Sensation, as of a splinter in the throat on swallowing. Belching accompanies most of the ailments.** Pulse irregular and intermittent. Palpitaion, wrose lying on the right side. Walks

and stands unsteadily. Great craving for sweets. Melancholic, apprehensive of some serious disease.

Potency —3rd to 30th and higher

17.   **Arjune**—A great heart remedy. Highly effective in cases of **high blood pressure,** with vertigo, palpitation and a sense of mental and physical exhaustion.

Potency —Lower potencies.

18.   **Arsenicum alb.**—**Great thirst, drinks much, but little at a time.** Nausea, retching and vomiting, after eating or drinking. Craves acids, coffee and pungent things. Heart-burn. Long-lasting eructations. **Is unable to lie down, fears suffocation. Palpitation.** Ascites and Anasarca. Abdomen painful and swollen, albuminous urine. Scanty and burning urine. great prostration. Gradual loss of weight from impaired nutrition. **Great anguish and restlessness. Despair drives him from place to place.**

Potency —3rd to 30th and higher

19.   **Asafoetida**—Syphilitic ulceration, with offensive, purulent discharges. Caries of different

bones. **Sensation of a ball rising in the throat. Flatulence. Great difficulty in bringing up the wind.** Cutting and burning in the stomach. Obstinate constipation. Spasmodic tightness in the chest, as if lungs could not be fully expanded.

Potency —2nd to 30th.

20. **Asparagus off.**—Its marked and immediate action on the urinary secretion is well-known. **Weakness and cardiac depression. Palpitation with oppression of the chest.** Great oppression in breathing. Rheumatic pain in the back, especially near shoulder and limbs.

Potency —6th to 30th.

21. **Aurum met.**—Hopeless, despondent, and great desire to commit suicide. **Palpitation and congestion. Is particularly useful for mercurio-syphilitic dyscrasia.** Peevish and vehement at least contradiction. Weakness of memory. Roaring in the head. **Violent headache. Congestion to head. Double vision; upper half of objects invisible. See fiery objects.** Horrible odor from the nose and mouth. Obstinate constipation. Stools hard and

painful. Urine turbid, like butter-milk. Dyspnea, worse at night. **Sleeplessness. Palpitation. Pulse rapid and irregular. Cardiac hypertrophy.** Arteriosclerosis with high blood pressure and nocturnal pain behind sternum. Tumultuous fluttering of heart and anxiety, with a sense of oppression in chest.

Also study **Aurum ars., Aurum brom., Aurum iod.** and **Aurum sulph.**

Potency—3rd to 30th. especially the latter.

22.   **Baryta carb.**—Sub-maxillary glands and tonsils enormously swollen. Takes cold easily. Can swallow only liquids. **Loss of memory. Irresolute. Lack of confidence in himself. Childish; grieves over trifles.** Great urging to urinate. Every time he attempts to urinate, his piles come down. Burning in the urethra on urinating. Suffocative cough. Fetid food-sweat. In **high blood pressure,** with Aneurism, Arteriosclerosis or Atheromatous condition of the blood-vessels, it is **a remedy par excellence.**

Also study **Baryta mur.**

Potency — 3rd to 30th and higher

23. **Belladonna**—It has a marked action on vascular system, skin and glands. Hence, **its complaints are always associated with hot, red skin flushed face, glaring eyes, throbbing carotids, excited mental states,** etc. Vertigo, with falling to the left side or backwards. Intense headache, worse from light, noise, jar, lying down and in afternoon; better by hard pressure and semi-erect posture. Constant moaning. Great thirst for cold water. Palpitation from least exertion.

    Potency —1st to 30th and higher.

24. **Benzoicum ac.**—Joints crack on motion. Rheumatic Gout, nodes very painful. Asthmatic cough, worse at night and from lying on right side. **Pain in the region of the heart. Brown and excessively bad-smelling urine.** Mental depression. Omits words in writing. Bowel movements mostly windy.

    Potency —3rd to 30th and higher.

25. **Bothrops lanc.**—Great lassitude and sluggishness. Hemiplegia with Aphasia. Nervous trembling. Face Puffy and swollen. Besotted expression. **Great difficulty of swallowing; cannot even swallow liquids.** Hemorrhages from

almost every orifice of the body. Black vomiting. Intense hematemesis.

Potency —6th to 30th.

26. **Bromium**—Every inspiration provokes cough. **Hypertrophy of the heart, from over-exercise or gymnastics. Difficult and painful breathing. Rattling of mucus in the larynx. Hoarseness. Testicles** swollen and indurated. Jerking and starting during sleep. Headache, worse from heat of sun and by rapid motion.

Potency —6th to 30th.

27. **Bryonia alb.**—Excessive dryness-of mucous membranes of the entire body, lips and tongue dry, hard, parched, cracked; stools dry, as if burnt; cough dry; racking. with scanty expectoration; urine dark and scanty. **GREAT THIRST, for large quantities at long intervals. Pressure, as from stone at pit of stomach, relieved by eructation** (*Nux vom., Pulsatilla*). Nausea and faintness when rising up. Mind exceedingly irritable. Everything puts him out of humor. Bursting headache, as if everything would be pressed out.

Potency —6th to 30th.

28. **Cactus grand.**—The whole body feels as if caged, each wire being twisted tighter. Atheromatous arteries with cardiac weakness. Oppressed breathing as from a weight on the chest. **Heart-constriction, as from an iron band. Angina pectoris, pain shooting down left arm. Palpitation, with vertigo, dyspnea and flatulence. Pulse irregular.** Screams with pain. Fear of death. Ill-humor. Congestive headache. Periodical head-pains, threatening Apoplexy. Blood vessels of the head distended. Profuse bleeding from the nose. **By its powerful action upon the heart and regularises the circulation, thereby dissipating acute congestion of head and chest, thus, bringing down the blood pressure.**

Potency —3rd to 20th.

29. **Calcarea ars.**—Violent rush of blood to head with vertigo. **Headache, better from lying on the painful side. Weekly headache. Albuminuria. Passes urine every hour. Slightest emotion causes palpitation.** Great

mental depression. Craving for alcohol. Complaints of fleshy women during menopause.

Potency —3rd to 200th.

30. **Calcarea carb.**—**Headache with cold** hands and feet. Vertigo, worse from ascending and when turning head. **Much perspiration over the head, wetting the pillow far around. Palpitation. Extreme dyspnea. Longing for fresh air. Incarcerated flatlence. Whitish, watery and sour-smelling stools.** Milk disagrees. Frequent sour eructations, or sour vomiting. Heart-burn. Troublesome cough at night, with free expectoration in the morning.

Potency —6th, 30th and higher.

31. **Cannabis ind.**—Chest oppressed with deep, labored breathing. Palpitation awakes him piercing pain in the cardiac region. **Sensation, as if the top of head were opening and shutting, or as if the calvarium were being lifted. Shocks through the brain.** Noises in the ear like boiling water. Constantly therorizing. Rapid change of mood. Excessive loquacity. Time seems too long, seconds seen ages.

Potency —Low attenuation to 200th.

32. **Carboneum sulph.**—Very useful in patients broken down by abuse of alcohol. Head aches, as from a tight cap. Ears feel obstructed. **Noise in the head. Changeable mood. Sluggishness. Arteries and veins congested.** Chronic rheumatism. Retinal congestion. Abdominal distension and rumbling.

    Potency —1st to 3rd, 30th and higher.

33. **Carbo veg.**—Excessive distension of the abdomen, worse after eating and drinking. **Gets temporary relief from belching. Rancid, sour or putrid eructations. Water-brash. Burning in the stomach. Slow digestion, food putrefies before it is digested. Cannot bear tigh clothing around waist and abdomen. Asthma, with blue skin and coldness in the extremities. Must be franned.** Offensive expectoration. Head feels heavy and constricted. Vertigo with nausea and tinnitus. Epistaxis in daily attacks.

    Potency —Low attenuation to 200th.

34. **Causticum**—Coryza with hoarseness. Paralysis of tongue, with indistinct speech. Gums bleed

readily. Acid dyspepsia. **Feels, as if lime were burned in the stomach. Urine expelled very slowly; sometimes retained. Cough with pain in the hip, and better by drinking cold water.** Pain in the chest with palpitation. Stiffness between shoulders. Paralysis of single parts. Unsteady walking. Aversion to sweets.

Potency —3rd to 30th and higher.

35. **Chelidonium maj.**—Small lumps of mucus fly from the mouth when coughing. **Feeling of constriction in the chest. Embarrassed respiration. Prefers hot food and drink.** Nausea or vomiting, better from taking very hot water. Gastralgia, relieved by eating pain through stomach to back and right shoulder-blade. **Right-sided headache. Fan-like motion of the alae nasi. Pain in the liver.** Hard stools, like sheep's dung. Clay-colored stools.

Potency —Lower attenuations to 200th.

36. **Chininum ars.**—Head feels too full. Throbbing headache. Vertigo, worse from looking up. Darting pain running up into head. Hyperchlorhydria. **Eggs produce diarrhea.**

Anorexia. Suffocative attacks, occurring in periodical periodical paroxysms. Must have open air. Palpitation. Sensation as if the heart stopped beating. Water taster bitter. Sleeplessness. Great irritability.

Potency —2nd and 3rd trits. to 200th.

37. **Cimicifuga rac.**—Irregular, trembling pulse. Angina pectoris. Numbness of the left arm; feels, as if bound to the side. **Heart's action ceases suddenly, impending suffocation. Rheumatic pains in muscles of back and neck. Pain from eyes to top of head. Waving sensation, or opening and shutting sensation in brain. Brain feels too large. Migraine.** Pain like electric shocks here and there. Sleeplessness, nausea and vomiting. Pain acros pelvis, from hip to hip.

Potency —3rd and higher to 30th.

38. **China off.**—Debility from exhausting discharges, from loss of vital fluids. **Sensation, as if skull would burst, or as if brain were balancing to and fro, and striking against skull. Intense throbbing of head and Carotids.** Scalp sensitive, wrose from combing

hair. Spots before eyes. Photophobia. Ringing in ears. Slow digestion. Tympanitic abdomen.

Potency —30th to 200th.

39. **Coca**—Useful in a variety of complaints incidental to mountain-climbing—such as, palpitation, dyspnea, anxiety and insomnia. Noises in ear. **Headache, with vertigo, preceded by flashes of light. Feeling, like a band across the forehead. Diplopia.** (*Gelsemium*). Longing for alcoholic liquors and tobacco. Short breath, especially in aged athletes and drunkards. Hemoptysis.

Potency —Tinct. to 3rd

40. **Coffea crud.**—Short, dry cough. Nervous palpittation. All senses are acutely sensitive. **Tossing about in anguish. Is full of ideas and quick to act. Seems, as if brain were torn to pieces, or as if nail were driven in head.** Intolerance of tight clothing about the stomach. Sleepless, on account of mental activity.

Potency —3rd to 200th.

41. **Conium mac.**—Sexual nervousness, with feeble erection. Testicles hard and enlarged. **Much**

difficulty in voiding urine; it flows and stops again. Frequent urging for stool. Tremulous weakness after every stool. Vertigo, when lying down and when turning over in bed. No inclination for business or study. Takes no interest in anything.

Potency —6th to 30th and higher.

42. **Convallaria maj.**—Dull headache. Coppery taste in the mouth. Tongue feels sore and scalded. Pain in the sacro-iliac joints, running down leg. **Orthopnea. Palpitation from least exertion. Tobacco heart, especially when due to cigarettes. Angina pectoris.** Extremely rapid and irregular pulse. Dropsy, due to heart troubles. Is of use when ventricles are over-distended and dilatation begins.

Potency —Tinct. 1 to 15 drops, and 3rd to 30th.

43. **Crataegus ony.**—It acts on the muscles of the heart and is a heart tonic. Myocarditis. Failing compensation. **Iregularity of heart. General Anasarca. Arteriosclerosis. Said to have a solvent power upon crustaceous and calcareous deposits in arteries.** Apprehensive and despondent. Air hunger. Dyspepsia. Irregular

pulse and breathing. Painful sensation of pressure in left side of chest below the clavicle. It is easpecially useful in LOW BLOOD PRESSURE, **with very feeble and irregular heart and pulse.** Great dyspnea on least exertion, palpitation and rapid action of the heart.

Potency —Mother Tinct.—5 drop doses, 2 or 3 times a day. Must be used for some time.

44. **Crotalus horr.**—Epistaxis. Vertigo, with weakness and trembling. Dull, heavy occipital pain, worse on right side and right eye. **Must walk on tip-toe to avoid jarring in the head. Great sadness. Clouded memory. Cannot lie on right side, without vomiting dark-green matter. Black or coffee-grounds vomiting.** Trembling, fluttering feeling below the epigastrium. Intestinal hemorrhage. Albuminous, scanty and dark-red urine. Cough, with bloody expectoration.

Potency —3rd to 6th, 30th and higher.

45. **Cuprum met.**—Face distorted, bluish and cyanotic. Contraction of the jaws, with foam at mouth. Constant protrusion and retraction of the tongue. **Stammering speech. Uses words**

not intended. Hiccough, preceding spasms. Strong metallic taste in mouth. When drinking, the fluid descends with a gurgling sound. Craving for cold drink. Spasmodic Asthma. Dyspnea with epigastric uneasiness. Angina pectoris, clonic spasms, beginning in fingers and toes with clenched thumbs.

Potency —6th to 30th.

46. Curare—Tired pain up and down the spine. Arms weak and heavy. Legs tremble; give way in walking. **Threatened paralysis of respiration on falling asleep. Short breath. Very distressing dyspnea.** Black spots before vision. Lancinating pains all over head. Nervous debility.

Potency —6th to 30th.

47. Digitalis pur.—Comes into play in all diseases where the heart is primarily involved. **The pulse is weak, irregular, intermittent or abnormally slow. Faintness and vomiting from motion. The least movement causes violent palpitation.** Sensation, as if the heart would stop beating, if he move (opposite to *Gelsemium*). Swelling of the feet. Cyanosis. Hydrocele,

scrotum enlarged like a bladder. Great weakness in chest, Cannot bear to talk.

Potency —3rd to 30th.

48. **Euphorbia lat.**—Labored breathing. Weak and fluttering heart's action. Pulse full, bounding and somewhat irregular. **Restlessness, worse at night. Sleep disturbed by anxious dreams.** Nausea and vomiting of copious, clear water, intermingled with white gelatinous lumps.

Potency —3rd to 30th.

49. **Fagopyrum**—Inability to study or to remember. Depressed and irritable. **Pain deep in head with upward pressure. Occipital headache. Pain around heart (better lying on back), extending of left shouder and arm.** Palpitation with oppression. Pulse irregular, intermittent or rapid. Drooling. Presistent morning nausea.

Potency —3rd and 12x.

50. **Ferrum met.** —**Voracious appetite or** absolute loss of appetite. Loathing of sour things. Eructation of food after eating. **Vomiting, immediately after eating. Vertigo on seeing flowing water. Hammering headache. Pain**

in back of head, with roaring in neck. Surging
of blood to chest. Palpitation, worse from
movement. Pulse full, but soft and yielding.
Dropsy, after loss of vital fluids.

Potency —3rd to 30th.

51.   **Ferrum phos.**—Its symptoms are more or less
corresponding to those of *Aconitum nap.* and
Belladonna. The typical Ferrum phos. subject is
rather full-blooded and robust, Rush of blood
to head, Ill-effects of sun-heat. **Throbbing
sensation in the head. Headache, better from
cold applications. Epistaxis, blood bright red.
Hemoptysis. Hard, dry cough with soreness
in the chest. Palpitation. Pulse rapid and
incompressible.** Articular rheumatism.
Rheumatic pain in shoulders. Face at times looks
flushed. Vomiting of undigested food.

Potency —3rd to 30th.

52.   **Gelsemium**—Great muscular weakness and
tired feeling. Dizziness, dullness and drowsiness.
General depression from heat of sun. Occipital
headache. **Band-like feeling around the head.
Wants to have the head raised on pillow.**

Double vision. Oppression about chest. Palpitation. Pulse slow when quiet, but greatly accelerated on motion. There is a feeling. as if it were necessary to keep the heart in motion, otherwise the heart's action would cease. As a rule, the Gels. patient has no thirst.

Potency —3rd to 200th.

53. **Glonoinum**—A great remedy for congestive head ache. Hyperemia of the brain, etc. Violent convulsions, associated with cerebral congestion. Surging of blood to head and heart. Confusion, with dizziness. Bad effects of sun-heat; sunstroke. Cannot recognize localities. Head feels enormously large, as if the skull were to small for the brain. Laborious action of the heart. Fluttering or palpitation, along with dyspnea. Cannot go uphill. Any exertion brings on rush of blood to heart and fainting spells. Throbbing in the whole body up to finger-tips. It is one of the best remedies for high blood pressure, having in its pathogenesis all the symptoms referable to a tendency to **sudden and violent irrgularities of the circulation, with surging of blood to the head and heart,**

violent bursting headache. etc., down to the full list.

Potency —6th to 30th and higher.

54. **Grindelia rob.**—An efficacious remedy for oppression and wheezing in bronchitic patients. The sibilant rales are disseminated with foamy mucus, very difficult to detach. **Asthma, with profuse, tenacious expectoration, which relieves. Breathing stops when falling asleep; wakes with a start and gasps for breath.** Must sit up in order to breathe. Cannot breathe when lying down. Cardiac weakness. From its frequent use, one can lower blood pressure.

Potency —Tinct. (1 to 15 drops) and the lower potenciss.

55. **Hydrastis can.**—Bronchitis in old, exhausted persons, with thick yellow tenacious expectoration. **Frequent fainting spells with cold sweat all over. Constipation. After stool, long-lasting pain in the rectum.** Anus fissured. Urine smells decomposed. Atonic dyspepsia. Tongue white, swollwn, large, flabby and slimy; shows imprint of teeth.

Potency —Tinct. to 30th.

56. **Hydrocyanic ac.**—Noisy and agitated breathing. Dry, spasmodic, suffocative cough. Venously congested lungs. **Marked cyanosis. Violent palpitation. Pulse weak and irregular. Extremities cold.** Torturing pain in the chest. Angina pectoris. Pain and tightness in the chest. Unconsciousness. Fears everything—horses, wagons, houses falling. etc.

    Potency —6th and higher.

57. **Iberis amar.**—Possesses great efficacy in cardiac diseases, since it has marked action upon the heart. Controls vascular excitement in hypertrophy with thickening of the heart's walls. Liver region full and painful. White stools. **Palpitation, with vertigo and choking in throat. Stitching pains in cardiac region. Pulse is full, irregular and intermitted. Worse from least motion and in a warm room.** Dropsy with enlarged heart. Violent palpitation induced by slightest exertion, or by laughing or coughing. Cardiac dyspnea. Tachycardia.

    Potency — Tinct. and 1st to 6th.

58. **Iodoformium**—Sharp, neuralgic pain in the head. Head feels heavy, as if it could not be lifted

from the pillow. **Feeling of a weight on the chest, as if smothering. Cough and wheezing on going to bed. Pain in the hert.** Hemoptysis. Asthmatic breathing. Abdomen distended. Chronic diarrhea. Temper irritable. Weakness of knees, when going upstairs.

Potency —Low trits.; 3rd to 30th.

59. **Kalium bich.**—Voice hoarse, worse evening. Metallic, hacking cough. Profuse, yellow expectoration, very glutinous and sticky, coming out in long, stringy and very tenacious mass. **Pain from mid-sternum to back. Cardiac dilatation, especially from co-existing renal lesion. Pains fly rapidly from one place to another.** Heavily coated tongue. Mapped tongue. Aphthae. Loaded feeling in the stomach immediately after eating. General weakness. Frontal headache.

Potency —3rd trit.; 6th and higher.

60. **Kalium carb.**—Drowsy after eating. Great exhaustion. Lumbago, with sharp pains extending up and down, back and to thighs. Cough, worse at 3a.m. **Leaning forword relieves chest symptoms. Palpitation and**

burning in the heart region. Sensation, as if heart were suspended. **Weak rapid or intermittent pulse.** Threatened heart-failure. Dropscial swelling of the extremities. Bag-like swelling of the upper eyelids. Involuntary urination when coughing. sneezing. etc. Sour vomiting. Easy choking when eating.

Potency —30th and higher; also 6th trit.

61. **Kalium phos.**—Paralytic numbness in back and extremities. Exertion aggravates. Breath offensive or fetid. Tongue coated brownish, like mustard. Spongy and receding gums. Cough with yellow expectoration. **Asthma, the least food aggravates. Shortness of breath, worse on going upstairs. Palpitation.** Vertigo worse when lying, sitting up or looking upward. Headache with weary, empty gone feeling in the stomach.

Potency —3rd to 12th trits.; 30th, 200th and higher.

62. **Kalmia lat.**—Gouty and rheumatic metastases to heart. Dyspnea. Shooting through chest above heart, into shoulder-blades. **Heart's action tumultuous, rapid and visible, Paroxysms of anguish around heart. Tachycrdia, with pain.**

Palpitation, worse from leaning forward. Fluttering of heart, with anxiety and mental depression. Bilious attacks with nausea, vertigo and headache. Joints red, hot and swollen.

Potency —Tinct. to 6th and higher.

63. **Lac can.**—Headache; pain first in one side, and then in the other. Blurred vision, nausea and vomiting, at the height of the attack of headache. **Dyspnea and palpitation. Throat feels raw, or burnt. Sorethroat; pain changing repeatedly from right to left, or vice versa.** Great hankering for pungent things. Great Lassitude. Sinking spells every morning. Spine very sensitive to touch or pressure.

Potency —30th to the highest.

64. **Lachesis nut.**—Gums swollen, spongy, bleeding easily. Tongue trembles, on attempting to protrude it, or catches on the teeth. Trifacial neuralgia, wrose on the left side. **Palpitation, with fainting spells, especially during climacteric. Constricted feeling in the chest. Irregular beating of the heart. Feel he must take a deep breath.** Cramp-like distress in the precordial region. Breathing almost stops, on

falling asleep. Hemorrhage from the bowels, like charred straw. Cannot bear anything around waist. General burning. Afflecting, as it does, the circulation, causing **rush of blood towards head, with coldness of feet, palpitation of heart, oppression of chest, inability to lie down, etc.,** Lachesis is well-adapted to cases of HIGH BLOOD PRESSURE, especially at the climacteric period of women.

Potency —6th to 200th. Not to be repeated too frequently.

65.   **Lithium carb.**—Turbid urine; mucus or red deposit in the urine. When urinating, pressure in the heart. **Rheumatic soreness in the cardiac region. Sudden shock in heart. Trembling and fluttering in heart, extending to back.** Constriction in chest. Violent cough, when lying down. Inspired air feels cold. Nodular swellings in the joints. Headache ceases while eating.

Potency —1st to 3rd trits, and up to the 200th.

66.   **Lycopodium clav.**—Deep furrows on forehead. Premature baldness and gray hair. Pressing headache on vertex, worse from 4 to 8 p.m. Dyspnea. **Tensive, constrictive, burning pain**

in chest. Aortic aneurism. Palpitation, worse at night or during the process of digestion. Cannot lie on the back, on account of suffocation. Burning between the scapulae. Pain in small of the back, before urinating; ceases after flow. Heavy, red sediment in the urine. Sour eructations. Desire for sweet things. Eating, even little, causes undue fullness in the stomach.

Potency —6th to 20th and higher.

67. **Lycopus virg.**—According to Dr. Hinsdale, it lowers blood pressure, reduces the rate of the heart, and increases the lenght of systole to a great degree. **Indiacated in diseases with tumultuous action of the heart and more or less pain. Hemoptysis, due to valvular heart disease. Precordial pain. Cyanosis.** Pulse weak, irregular or intermittent. Frontal headache. Supra-orbital pain, with aching in testicles. Nosebleed.

Potency—1st to 30th and higher.

68. **Magnesium carb.**—Bursting headache; worse from motion or open air, and better from pressure, or wrapping up warmly. Much sweating

of head. **Palpitation and cardiac pain, while sitting; better by moving about** (*Gelsemium*). **Stools knotty, like sheep's dung, crumbling at verge of anus.** Painful, smarting hemorrhoids. Liver enlarged. Bloating of the abdomen. Urine can only be passed by pressing abdominal muscles. Anxious dreams with restless sleep.

potency —Tinct. (5 drops) 30th to 200th.

70.   **Magnesium phos.**—Cramps in calves. General muscular weakness. Bloated or full sensation in abdomen. Must loosen clothing. Walk about and constantly pass flatus. **Asthmatic oppression of chest. Spasmodic cough. Nervous palpitation. Angina Pectoris. Constricting pains around heart.** Flatulent colic, forcing the patient to bend double. Hiccough, with retching, day and night. Supra-orbital pains, worse, right side.

Potency —1st to 12th; sometimes the highest are preferable.

71.   **Magnolia grand.**—Rheumatism and cardiac lesions are prominent features in the symptomatology of this drug. Alternating pains,

between spleen and heart. **Suffocated feeling, when walking fast, or lying on left side. Dyspnea. Crampy pain in heart. Angina pectoris. Tendency to faint away. Sensation, as if the heart head stopped beating. Pain around heart.** Numbness in left arm. Erratic shifting of pains. Itching of the feet.

Potency—3rd to 30th.

72. **Medorrhinum**—Much oppression of breathing. Incessant, dry, night cough. **Asthma. Can inhale, but cannot exhale** (*Sambucus*). **Cough, better from lying on stomach. Burning of hands and feet.** Heels and balls of feet tender. Soreness of soles. Headache from jarring of cars, exhaustion or hard work. Gleety discharge; the whole urethra feels sore. Sleeps in knee-chest position.

Potency —Highest. Not to be repeated often.

73. **Melilotus all.**—Violent, congestive headache with intense redness and flushing of the face. Throbbing of the carotids. **Profuse epistaxis. Feels, as if smothering, especially from rapid walking. Hemoptysis.** Sensation of a heavy

weight upon the chest. No desire for stool, until there is a large accumulation (*Bryonia, Alumina*).

Potency —Lower;. or up to the 30th.

74. **Moschus—Fainting fits, convulsious, catalepsy, pressure on the top of the head. Vertigo, worse from least motion.** Sensation as if falling from a great height. Premature senility. Impotence, associated with Diabetes. Violent sexual desire.

Potency —1st to 3rd and 30th.

75. **Muriaticum ac.** —Hemorrhoids, with great sensitiveness to touch; even sheet of toilet paper is painful. Cannot bear the sight or tought of meat. Fetid breath. Deep ulcers on tongue. **Heart intermits every third beat. Pulse rapid, feeble and small.** Cannot urinate without having bowels move at the same time. Tottering gaits. Excessive prostration.

Potency —1st to 3rd; 30th and higher.

76. **Naja trip.**—Its action settles around heart, hence, it is almost a specific for a variety of cardiac complaints, arising from hypertrophy and valvular lesions. With heart symptoms, there is

apt to be pain in the forehead and temples. Suicidal mania. Severe mental depression. Aversion to talking. Palpitation. Stitching pain in the region of the heart. Angina pectoris. Pulse slow, weak and irregular. Sleeps with stertorous breathing. Grasping at throat, with sense of choking. Irritating, dry cough, dependent on cardiac lesions. Asthmatic constriction, worse in the evening.

Potency —6th to 30th.

77. **Natrium mur.**—Irritable. Gets into a passion about trifles. **Consolation aggravates. Headache, as if a thousand little hammers were knocking on the brain. Chronic headache, from sunrise to sunset. Fluttering or palpitation of the heart. Heart's pulsation shake the body. Heart intermits on lying down.** Cough, with bursting pain in head. Shortness of breath, especially on going upstairs. Has to wait a long time, before the urine is passed. Unquenchable thirst.

Potency—12th to 30th and higher.

78. **Natrium sulph.**—Edema of feet. Pain in the limbs, compelling him frequently to change his

position. Thick, greenish discharge from the urethra. **Dyspnea, worse during damp weather. Cough with thick, ropy, greenish expectoration. Constant desire to take deep, long breath. Palpitation. Pain through lower left chest.** Loose morning stools. Liver region sore to touch. Cannot bear tight clothing around waist. Flatulency; wind colic. Rumbling in the abdomen.

Potency —1st to 12th trits.

79. **Nux vom.**—It is the greatest of all polychrests, because bulk of its symptoms correspond with those of the commonest diseases. Frontal headache. Congestion in the brain. Head feels distended. Photophobia; much worse in the morning. **Oppressed breathing, expecially after eating. Shallow respiration. Cough brings on bursting headache and bruised pain in the epigastrium. Nervous palpitation. Bad effects of sexual excesses.** Spermatorrhea with weakness, backache and irritability. Liver engorged, with stitches and soreness. Difficult belching. Wants to vomit, but often fails. Frequent, ineffectuall urging for stool. Incomplete and unsatisfactory stools.

Potency —1st to 30th and higher.

80. **Opium**—Feces protrude and recede (*Silicea, Thuja*). Obstinate constipation. Severe colic, with passage of round, hard, black balls like stool. Breathing stops, on going to sleep. **Deep snoring or rattling breathing. Complete loos of consciousness. Apoplexy. Thinks he is not at home. Bursting feeling in the head.** Face looks red and swollen or dark red, lower jaw hanging down. Pupils insensible to light. Urine retained or passes involuntarily. Full and slow pulse.

Potency —3rd to 200th and higher.

81. **Oxalicum ac.**—Complaints are made worse when thinking of them. Palpitation with dyspnea. **Angina pectoris. Sharp, lancinating pain in the left lung, coming on suddenly, depriving of breath. Precordial pains dart to the left shoulder.** Aortic insufficiency. Hoarseness or aphonia. Testicles feel contused and heavy. Easy sweating. Muscular prostration. Backache.

Potency —6th to 30th.

82. **Paris quad.**—Soreness on the top of the head; hence, he cannot brush hair. Occipital headache. **Head feels large and expanded. Constant**

hawking, on account of viscid, green mucus in larynx and trachea. Sense of weight and weariness in nape of neck and across shoulders. Sensation of a string through eyeballs.

Potency —3rd to 30th.

83.   **Petroleum**—Must rise at night and eat; Diabetes. Epistaxis. Nostrils ulcerated. Eczema, intertrigo, etc. in and behind the ears with intense itching. Herpetic eruptions on the perineum. **Cough produces headache. Oppression of the chest, worse at night. Sensation of coldness in the region of the heart. Palpitation. Fainting with ebullitions, heat, etc.** Fetid sweat in axillae. Knees stiff. Cracking in joints. Rhagades, worse in winter. Low spirited, with dimness of sight. Loses his way in streets.

Potency —3rd to 30th and higher.

84.   **Phosphoricum ac.**—Heavy and confused feeling in the head. Crushing headache. Cannot collect his thoughts or find the right word. Memory impaired. **Frequent flow of urine. Polyuria, worse at night. Sexual power deficient. Scrotal eczema. Difficult**

respiration. Weak feeling in chest, worse from talking. Pressure behind the sternum, rendering obstruction in breathing. Palpitation. Pulse irregular or intermittent. Craves juicy or pungent things. Shows dislike for sour or acid substances. Distension and fermentation in the bowels.

Potency —1st to 200th.

85. Phosphorus —Vertigo, worse after rising. Heat comes from the spine. Patient is restless and fidgety. Loss of memory. Oversensitive to external impressions. Vexed easily. Cough from tickling in the throat. Feels tightness across the chest or sensation of great weight on the chest. Repeated hemoptysis. Violent palpitation, worse lying on left side. Heart dilated, especially the right chambers. Feeling of warmth in the heart. Lack of sexual power, although there is irresistible desire. Involuntary emissions, with lascivious dreams. Constipation. Stools narrow and long, like a dog's; difficult to expel. Burning sensation in the palms and soles.

Potency —3rd to 200th and higher. Not to be repeated continuously.

86.   **Physostigma vene.**—Constant pain on the top
      of the head. Pain over orbits; cannot bear to raise
      eyelids. Feeling as if a ball came up to the throat.
      **Palpitation. Spasmodic action of the heart,
      with feeling of pulsation through the whole
      body. Beats of heart distinctly perceptible in
      the head and chest. Fluttering of the heart
      felt in the throat.** Numbness of the hands and
      feet. Sudden jerking of limbs, on going to sleep.
      Chronic constipation.

      Potency —3rd to 30th.

87.   **Phytolacca dec.**—Ulcerated sore-throat. Tonsils
      and fauces swollen, with burning pain, cannot
      swallow even water. **Feeling, as if heart leaped
      into throat. Shocks of pain in the cardiac
      region, alternating with pain in the right
      arm.** Syphilitic bone-pains. Chronic
      rheumatism. Aching, soreness and restlessness.
      Constipation of the aged. Painful induration of
      testicles. Shooting along perineum to penis.

      Potency —3rd to 200th.

88.   **Plumbum met.**— Hypertension and
      arteriosclerosis. Excessive and rapid emaciation.
      Loss of memory. Slow perception. Amnesic

aphasia. Paretic dementia. Face looks pale and cachectic; cheeks sunken. **Cardiac weakness. Palpitation. Wiry pulse, soft and small pulse. Paralysis of the lower extermities, as a result of Apoplexy.** Albuminous urine. chronic interstitial nephritis with scanty urine. Excessive colic radiating to all parts of the body. Obstructed evacuation from impaction of feces.

Potency —3rd to 200th and higher.

89. **Pulsatilla**—Averse to fat and warm food and drink. Heart-burn. Thirstlessness. Vomiting of food eaten long before. Pressure as from a stone in the abdomen; must loosen clothing. **Cough, with thick, bland and easy expectoration. Short breath; anxiety and palpitation, when lying on the left side. Smothering sensation on lying down.** Wakes languid and unrefreshed. Intolerable burning heat at night, with distended veins. Heat in one part of body with coldness in others. One-sided sweat. Longing for open air.

Potency —3rd to 200th and higher.

90. **Pyrogenium**—Bursting headache, with restlessness, horribly offensive breath.

Constipation, with complete inertia of the rectum. Large, black and carrion-like stools. **Cardiac asthenia, from septic conditions. Distinct consciousness of a heart. The heart feels tired or it feels as if enlarged. Constant purring, throbbing or pulsating in the ears, preventing sleep.** *Pulse abnormally rapid—out of all proportion to temperature, great restlessness; must move constantly, to relieve the soreness of the parts affected.* It is to be given when the best-selected remedy fails to relieve or permanently improve.

Potency —6th to 200th and higher. Not to be repeated frequently.

91.   **Rhus tox.**—Pain between shoulders, on swallowing. Hot, painful swelling of joints. Dark, turbid and high-colored urine. Lumbago. **Triangular redness at the tip of the tongue. Fever-blisters around mouth. Want of appetite. Desire for milk. Bronchial cough, worse on awaking, with expectoration of small plugs of mucus cardiac hypertrophy from over-exertion.** Quick, weak, irregular or intermittent pulse with numbness of left arm.

Trembling and palpitation, when sitting still. Nose-bleed on stooping.

Potency —6th to 200th and higher.

92. **Rowalfia serp.**—This drug has come to the fore only very recently and has started snatching laurels in cases of high blood pressure in its various degree of intensity and acuteness. It has been credited with quickly softening the action of the heart, thereby normalising the circulation, dissipating the violent congestion of head and heart thus, tending to bring the blood pressure down, even from a frightening level. The **violent congestion, bursting, throbbing headache and tumultuous throbbing of the temporal arteries quickly subside, hemorrhages from nose or from somewhere else quickly stops, giddiness vanishes, normal sleep is restored and the patient soon feels tranquillity of body and mind.** The drug has not yet been proved upon the healthy and in homeopathic words, it is being used only clinically. From its clinical reports it is obvious that it can be compared with *Acon nap., Belladonna, Cactus, Glonoine, Sulphur,* etc. in combating high blood pressure.

Potency —Alcoholic Tinct.—8 to 10 drop, doses– 2 or 3 times a day or more.

93. Sanguinaria can.—Face looks flushed. Periodical sick headache. Pain begins in occiput, spreads upwards, and settles over eyes—especially right. Chronic rhinitis. Craving for piquant things. Unquenchable thirst. **Cough of gastric orgin, relieved by eructation. Offensive breath and expectortion. Asthma, with stomach disorders. Palpitation, worse from exertion.** Climacteric ailments with excessive burning, especially in the palms and soles. Rheumatism of right shoulder. It is adapted to high blood pressure, especially of the females at climaxis, characterized by **flushes of heat with circumscribed redness of the cheeks, detrmination of blood to head and chest, distension of temporal veins, burning of palms and soles, the characteristic occipital headache, etc.**

Potency —6th to 200th.

94. **Secale cor.**—Icy-coldness of the extremities. Fingers and feet bluish, shrivelled and bent backwards. Putrid discharges. **Dyspnea and**

cardiac oppression, with cramp in the diaphragm. Precordial tenderness. Palpitation, with contracted and intermittent pulse. Unquenchable thirst. Burning in the stomach or abdomen. The skin feels cold to the touch, yet the patient cannot tolerate covering. Burning in all parts of the body, as if sparks of fire were falling on the patient (*Arsenic alb.*).

Potency —6th to 200th.

95. **Sepia off.**—Yellowish saddle across the nose. Headache in terrible shocks at menstrual nisus, with scanty flow. **Prodromal symptoms of Apoplexy. Fullness in the rectum. Disposition to vomit after eating. Constipation. Bleeding at stool. Dark-brown, round balls are passed with great difficulty. Violent palpitation. Beating in all arteries. Tremulous feeling, with flushes of heat.** Oppression of chest, especially in the evening. Dyspnea, better from rapid motion. Cough with profuse, salty expectoration in the morning. Burning on the vertex, in the eyes, plams and soles.

Potency —12th, 200th and higher, Not to be repeated too frequenty.

96. **Silicea**—Great sensitiveness to taking cold Prostration of mind and body. Brain-fag, nervous and excitable. Headache. **Pains begin in occiput, spreads over head and settles over eyes. Profuse sweating, especially on the head. Cough with muco-purulent expectoration.** Rectum feels paralysed. Stools come down with difficulty. When partly expelled, they recede again. Want of appetite. Excessive thirst. Disgust for meat and warm food. Sour eructations, after eating. Offensive sweat on hands, feet and axillae.

    Potency —6th to 200th and higher.

97. **Spartium scop.**—It increases the strength of the heart, slow it, and reduces the blood pressure. It continues the good effects of *Veratrum* and *Digitalis,* without any of the undesirable effects of either (Hinsdale). From its action, the total amount of urine is also increased. The drug has, therefore, diuretic properties, and is useful in dropsy, albuminuria, with arterial hypertension or Arteriosclerosis.

    Potency—1st to 3rd trits.

98. **Spigelia anth.**—Semi-lateral headache, involving the left eye. Violent, throbbing

headache, worse from making a false step. **Violent palpitation. Frequent attacks of palpitation, which is quite audible and visible from a distance. Rheumatic carditis. Pulse weak and irregular. Dyspnea, must lie on the right side, with head high.** Frequent, ineffectual urging to stool. Severe pain in and around eyes, extending deep into socket. Ciliary neuralgia or prosopalgia. Sun headache.

Potency —2nd to 200th.

99. **Spongia tosta**—Barking cough, worse before midnight. Short panting breathing. Cough abates after eating or drinking especially warm drinks. It also relieves the dry, sympathetic, chronic cough of organic heart disease (*Naja*). Chest weak, can scarcely talk. **Rapid and violent palpitation, with dyspnea, cannot lie down. Awakens suddenly after midnight, with pain and suffocation; is flushed, hot and frightened to death.** (*Aconitum nap.*). **Valvular insufficiency. Angina pectoris with faintess and anxious sweat.** Ebullitions of blood, viens distened. Cardiac hypertophy, especially the right, with asthmatic symptoms. Swelling of the

spermatic cords and testicles.

Potency —3rd to 200th.

100. **Sticta pulm.**—Dull headache with heavy pressure in the forehead and root of the nose. Rheumatic stiffness of the neck. **Dryness of the nasal mucous membrane. Constant need to blow the nose, but no discharge. Dry scabs, especially in the evening and night. Incessant sneezing. Dropping of mucus posteriorly. Dry hacking cough during night, wrose from inspiration.** Pulsation from right side of sternum down to abdomen. Swelling, heat and redness of joints.

Potency —6th to 200th.

101. **Stramonium**—The entire force of this drug seems to be expended on the brain. Loquacity. Violent and lewd. Cannot bear solitude or darkness. **Rush of blood to the head. Staggers, with tendency to fall forward and to the left. Eyes seem prominet. Pupils dilated. Loss of vision or double vision. Hot circumscribed redness of cheeks. Blood rushes to face.** Violent thirst. Vomiting of mucus and green bile. Urine almost suppressed. Sexual erethism, with

indecent speech and action. Sleepy, but cannot sleep. Awakenens terrified. Profuse sweat, which does not relieve.

Potency—30th and higher.

102. **Strophantus hisp.**—It acts on the heart, increasing the systole and diminishing the rapidity. May be use with advantage to tone the heart and run off dropsical accumulations. **Anemia, with palpitation and breathlessness. Arteriosclerosis, rigid arteris of the aged. Irritable heart of tobacco smokers. Scanty and albuminous urine. Temporal headache, with double vision.** Extremities swollen. Dropsical condition. Edema of lungs. "*Strophanthus,* occasions no gastric distress, has no cumulative effects, is a greater diuretic, and is safer for the aged."

Potency —Tinct. and 6th.

103. **Strychninum pur.**—Bursting headache. Vertigo, with roaring in the ears. Sparks before eyes. Deglutition impossible. Joints stiffened. **Constant retching with violent vomiting. Griping pain in the bowels. Very obstinate constipation. Fluttering sensation in the**

cardiac region. **Cardiac asthma.** Perspiration, in a stream down head and chest. Lower extremities turn cold. Cramp-like pains. Spasms, provoked by the slightest touch and attempt to move). Tetanic convulsion.

Potency —3rd to 30th.

104. **Sulfonalum**—Constant desire to urinate. Scanty brownish-red urine. Albuminuria, with tube-casts. Pulmonary congestion. Stertorous breathing. Sighing, **dyspnea. Vertigo. Double vision. Profound weakness Mental confusion. Incoherency. Extreme irritability.** Legs seem too heavy. Staggering gait. Muscular twitchings. Sleeplessness or drowsiness. Extreme restlessness.

Potency —3rd trit.

105. **Sulphur**—Constant heat on the top of the head. Beating headache, with vertigo, worse from stooping. Heat and burning in the eyes. Bitter taste, especially in the morning. **Great acidity - sour eructation. Drinks much, eats little. Difficult respiration. Wants windows open. Heat throughout chest. Flushes of heat in chest, rising to head. Palpitation.** Frequent

micturition, especially at night. Must hurry–
sudden call to urinate. Hard, knotty, insufficient
stools. Cat-naps, slightest noise awakens.
Unhealthy skin; every little injury suppurates,
Itching of the genitals, when going to bed.

Potency —Lowest to highest.

106. **Sumbulus mos.**—Choking constriction;
constant swallowing. Belching of gas from
stomach. Tenacious mucus in the throat.
**Abdomen full, distended and painful
Climacteric flushes. Nervous palpitation.
Loses breath on any exertion. Irregular pulse.**
Insomnia, feels dull in the morning. Mistakes in
writing and adding. Oily pellicle on the surface
of the urine.

Potency — tinct. to 3rd.

107. **Tabacum**—Violent constriction of the chest.
Precordial oppression, with palpittion and pain
between shoulders. **Dyspnea, nausea and
vomiting terrible, faint, sinking feeling at the
pit of the stomach. Wants abdomen
uncovered. It lessen nausea and vomiting.
Hiccough. Tachycardia or bradycardia.**

Hands and legs icy-cold. Shufling or unsteady gait. Paralysis, folowing Apoplexy. Copious, drenching sweat, sweat with giddiness. Intermittent pulse.

Potency —3rd to 30th and higher.

108. **Tarantula hisp.**—Extreme restlessness; must keep in constnt motion. Destructive impulses; moral relaxation. Vertigo. Intense pain in the head. Sensation, as if thousands of needles were pricking into brain. **Palpitation. Precordial anguish. Sensation, as if heart twisted and turned around.** Twitching and jerking of the extremities. Numbness of the legs. spinal irritation. Choreic movements. Profuse menstruation, with frequent erotic spasms.

Potency —6th to 200th.

109. **Terebinthinae ol.**—Vertigo, with vanishing of vision. Feeling, like a band around the head. Dry, red, sore or shining tongue. **Choking sensation in the throat. Stomatitis. Strangury, with bloody urine. Constant tenesmus.**

Intense burning in the hypogastric region. Scanty or suppressed urine. Watery, greenish or bloody stools. Difficult breathing. Rapid, small, thready or intermittent pulse.

Potency —1st to 200th.

110. **Thea chin.**—Sinking sensation at epigastrium, or faint, gone feeling in the stomach. Craving for acids. Dyspepsia. **Sudden production of gas in considerable quantities. Borborygmus. Anxious opression. Precordial anguish. Palpitation. Unable to lie on the left. side. Rapid, irregular or intermittent pulse. Sleepless** at night, with vascular excitement and restlessness. Horrible dreams. Hallucination of 'hearing. Ill-humour. Congestive headache. Sick headache, radiating from one point.

Potency —3rd to 30th.

111. **Theridion cura.**—Restlessness, finds pleasure in nothing. Time passes too quickly. Headache, worse when any one is walking over the floor. **Is sensitive to noise; it penetrates the body, especially teeth. Pressure behind eyeballs. Throbbing over left eye. Nausea and vomiting, worse when closing the eyes and on motion. Luminous vibration before eyes.**

Pinching in the left pectoral muscles. **Cardiac anxiety and pain.** Burning in the liver region. Sensitiveness between vertebrae. Avoids pressure on spine.

Potency —6th and 30th

112. **Thyroidinum**—Irritable; goes into a rage over a trifle. Frontal headache, with a flushed face. Tongue thickly coated. Polyuria. Presence of sugar or albumen in the urine. Dry, painful cough, with scanty and difficult expectoration. **Anxiety about chest, as if constricted. Palpitation from least exertion. Sever heart pain. Ready excitablity of heart. Tachycardia** (Naja) **Cardiac oppression, with inability to lie down.** Weak, frequent pulse. Sensation of faintness and nausea. Edema of legs. Jaundice, with pruritus. Amblyopia. Goitre.

Potency —6th to 30th.

113. **Uranium nit.**—Burning pain in the stomach. Abdomen bloated. Excessive thirst, nausea and vomiting. **Ravenous appetite. Copious urination. Incontinence of urine. Diabetes, burning in the urethra, with very acid urine.**

Rapid emaciation and debility. Tendency to Ascites and general Dropsy. Degeneration of the liver, with high blood pressure and edema.

Potency —2nd trit. to 6th trit.

114. **Valeriana off.** —Changeable disposition. Over-sensitiveness. Feeling of intoxication. Sensation, as of a thread hanging down throat. Foul eructations. **Heartburn, with gulping up of rancid fluid. Nausea, with faintness. Choking on falling asleep. Spasmodic asthma.** Rheumatic pains in limbs. Pain in the heels, when sitting. Sciatica, pain worse on standing and resting on floor.

Potency —Tinct.; 6th to 200th.

115. **Veratrum alb.**—Sits in a stupid manner; notices nothing. Sullen indifference. Frenzy of excitement; shrieks and curses. Aimless wandering from home. Headache, with nausea and vomiting. **Face very pale, blue, collapsed or cold. Cold sweat on forehead, with difficulty of breathing and rattling in the chest.** Palpitation, with anxiety and rapid, audible respiration. Irregular, feeble or intermittent

pulse. Heart disease, arising from excessive use of tobacco. Giddiness, with sunken features and icy-coldness. Craves fruits, ice, juicy fruits and cold things. Great weakness, after purging and vomiting. Thirst for cold water. Averse to warm food.

Potency —1st to 200th.

116. **Veratum vir.**—Especially adapted to fullblooded and plethoric persons. **Intense congestion in the head with blood-shot eyes. Sun-stroke. Flushed face.** Convulsive twitching of facial muscles. Headache starts from the nape of the neck; cannot hold up the head. Nausea, retching and vomiting. Smallest quantity of food or drink is immediately rejected. Hiccough. Scanty flow of urine, with cloudy sediment, **Constant, dull, burning pain in the region of the heart. Valvular diseases of the heart. Pulse may be slow, soft, weak, irregular or intermittent.** Congestion, especially to lungs, or base of the brain. Rheumatism of heart. Quarrelsome and delirious.

Potency—1st to 6th.

117. **Viscum alb.**—Burning and stopped up feeling in the ear. Double vision. Feeling as if the whole vault of the skull were lifted up. Dyspnea. **Feeling of suffocation, when lying on the left side. Stertorous breathing. Spasmodic cough. Arterial hypertension with valvular insufficiency. Unable to rest in a reclining position.** Edematous swelling of the extremities. A glow seems to rise from the feet to the head— seems to be on fire. General tremor. Climacteric complaints.

Potency —Tinct.; 3x to 200th.

118. **Xanthophylum**—Hemiplegia, or anterior crural neuralgia. Neuralgic shooting pain, as from electricity; all over limbs. **Occipital headache. Weight and pain on vertex. Constant desire to take a long breath. Oppression of chest. Dry cough, day and night.** Dysentery, with tympanites and tenesmus. Sleeplessness. Mental depression. Nervousness. Easily frightened, Painful hemorrhages.

Potency —1st to 30th.

119. **Zincum met.**—Soles of feet sensitive. Steps with entire sole of foot on floor. Varicose veins on

legs, etc. Feet in continued motion; cannot keep them still. Vertigo; feels as if he would fall to the left side. **Headache, worse from the smallest quantity of wine. Rolls the head from side to side or bores the head into the pillow. Occipital pain, with weight on vertex. Bronchitis, with constriction of the chest. Dyspnea; better as soon as expectoration appears. Palpitation.** Retention of urine; can only void urine when sitting bent backwards. Flatulent colic. Liver enlarged and indurated. Hard and small stool; passed with great difficulty. Pain in small of the back.

Potency —6th to 200 and higher.

VII. Resume of the Therapeutics of Blood Pressure

In emergent cases of high blood pressure, quick reduction of the pressure is the main task.

What is needed in such cases is that the remedy must have the power to lower the blood pressure by softening the action of the heart quickly and to equalise the circulation to relieve the surging of blood to the head and heart and thus quiet down the violent congestive, bursting headache. The tumultuous throbbing of the distended temporal arteries etc. down the whole list, thereby inducing normal sleep with peace and tranquility of the body and mind.

This may be effected by a judicial application of medicines like **Cactus grand, Glonoine, Rowvolfia, Amyl nit, Lycopus, Spartium scop, Arjun,** etc. ranking the highest. Among others may be mentioned **Aconitum nap, Belladonna, Crataegus, Kalium phos, Digitalis pur, Convallaria maj,** etc which have also proved of much value in suitable cases.

For high blood pressure with Arteriosclerosis or Atheromatus condition of the blood-vessels the most effective remedies are **Adrenalin, Baryta Carb, the Aurums, Plumbum, Strophanthus** etc. For Blood Pressure with Pulmonary lesions—**Phosphorus.** For blood pressure at the climacteri—**Glonoine, Sanguinaria, Lachesis, Sepia, Cactus,** etc.

For **low-blood pressure,** the most credited remedies are **Gelsemium, Baryta Carb, Conjum, Crataegus, Adrenalin, China off, Carbo veg.** and some others.

Of course, a careful study of all the remedies as treated in the text will pay rich dividends in both types of blood pressures.

A strict observance of the dietary, as mentioned in the text for such cases is, of paramount importance. To speak in short, the diet of subjects of high blood pressure must be lower than normal, with strict control of the intake of salty foods; and the diet for subjects of low blood pressure should be just the opposite and as much nourishing as suits the digestive capacity of the patients.

– The End –